I0458297

HOW I UNLEARNED
MY CRAP

MY PERSONAL STORY
BOOK II

KATHY BALDWIN
AWARD-WINNING AUTHOR

© 2025 ALL RIGHTS RESERVED.

Published by She Rises Studios Publishing **www.SheRisesStudios.com.**

No part of this book may be reproduced or transmitted in any form whatsoever, electronic, or mechanical, including photocopying, recording, or by any informational storage or retrieval system without the expressed written, dated and signed permission from the publisher and author.

LIMITS OF LIABILITY/DISCLAIMER OF WARRANTY:

The author and publisher of this book have used their best efforts in preparing this material. While every attempt has been made to verify the information provided in this book, neither the author nor the publisher assumes any responsibility for any errors, omissions, or inaccuracies.

The author and publisher make no representation or warranties with respect to the accuracy, applicability, or completeness of the contents of this book. They disclaim any warranties (expressed or implied), merchantability, or for any purpose. The author and publisher shall in no event be held liable for any loss or other damages, including but not limited to special, incidental, consequential, or other damages.

ISBN: 978-1-966798-07-1

Dedication

To those who dare to unlearn and level up beyond the confines of their past. This book is a testament to the power within each of us to transform, guided by the universal truths that connect us all. May it inspire you to embrace your journey with courage and grace.

To the four generations of women in my family—from my grandmothers to my mother and my daughter. We carry the weight of past generations, and with it, the heartbreaks and challenges that have shaped our paths. Yet, through the trials and the unlearning of inherited burdens, my love for each of you remains deep and profound. You live in my heart and soul daily, shaping me into who I am. Your stories and contributions to my journey of unlearning cannot be acknowledged enough. It is through your strength and wisdom that I find my own, and for that, I am eternally grateful.

Table of Contents

Acknowledgments

I extend my deepest gratitude to She Rises Studios and the entire team. Your belief in me and dedication to bringing my books to life have been invaluable. Having a publisher who knows me personally and works tirelessly behind the scenes means the world to me. This is what publishing should be.

An extra special thanks to Hanna Olivas. You have become my friend and mentor, my Gayle. Through your vision and passion, I am finding my alignment and understanding what it truly means when women support women. I believe in universal timing, and having this book released alongside our collaboration with She Wins Women's Networking Group shows me the magic, power and synergy of the divine feminine.

To my advance reading team and editors—Marcy Bialeschki, Heather Hansen, and Devin Sarno—thank you for your insights, observations, and wisdom. This book is deeper and more intimate because of your contributions.

To my dear friend Kim Beam, your friendship and encouragement have been a guiding light. Thank you for spending time over video reading this with me and allowing me to see the book through the eyes of the reader. I am eternally grateful to the universe for bringing us together.

A special thank you to Raimonda Jan for pushing me to my limits. You are the reason I recognize the need to constantly level up and own my place. Never stop challenging your clients with such deep, profound love.

To my family and friends, thank you for challenging me to see my crap and rise above it. Seeing myself through you has allowed me to find my own personal alignment, even and especially when it was painful. I believe that it will all be worth it in the end.

Lastly, to Rick Roy, none of this would be possible without your belief in me and unwavering support.

Before I Begin...

Welcome to How I Unlearned MY Crap. This book is the follow-up to **"Unlearn the Crap and Level UP: Your Soul is Calling"**.

That book was all the lessons that I learned and the path and knowledge to how you can unlearn your own crap. This book, How I Unlearned my Crap, is the why and how the crap was created for me. It is my root cause analysis.

This book is an intimate conversation where I invite you into my world and share with you my vulnerable deepest secrets, pains, and traumas. For those of you who have your own traumas please be prepared, you will probably be triggered. I want you to know that if you're triggered by anything that I've experienced, it is your soul showing you where you have crap that needs to be released. It is your soul's language. It is your mirror. Everything we feel, see, think and experience is a direct communication from our inner self to our conscious self. I invite you to lean into those triggers. That is where your power lies.

This book is a conversation between you and me as if we were sitting on my couch together sharing a glass of wine or cup of tea or as a dear friend of mine would choose a cup of hot water. It is me with an open heart sharing for the purpose of serving.

My style of writing is unique and I hope it's not confusing to you. I have taken multiple moments in time and connected them to the universal law of cause and effect. My goal is to show how the neuroplasticity of our brain takes an initial thought and belief and then looks for proof that it's right because our brains are wired to always be right.

That proof of being right allows our brain to deepen those neural pathways and creates disempowering cycles, and just like that process creates crap in our brain we can also use the same process to unlearn the crap and create pathways that are empowering.

I write as if I'm talking to you because that's what I believe I'm doing. I'm opening my heart, my soul and allowing you to see your own crap through my journey.

My goal is that these stories are not trauma vomiting but instead insights into how we can discern the patterns, find the root causes and unlearn anything that is disempowering.

I want you to know that the title Unlearn the Crap was not a marketing ploy. The word crap was not anything that I had used before. All of this was born out and through my breakdown. When I had my complete and total breakdown I was immediately filled with these epiphanies, these words, these insights. It was as if I had full clarity and vision. It was the beauty of my healing and transformation that happened since I wrote my first book. The proof of what I was saying and thinking and feeling was everywhere. The things that I did not see before while I was locked in my patterns, suddenly appeared before me. Synchronicities happened. Awakenings happened. My empowerment happened.

Crap is excrement. It is physical. It is the process of eliminating that which doesn't serve us. It is also the trauma responses that have been suppressed, that have been turned into inflammation by holding on to the cortisol and the stress and the hormones. It is physical in the way that our body uses our lymphatic system and our fascia to hold and/or release the traumas and the disempowerment. It is physical in that it affects our gut microbiome. It is physical in how it creates disease and pain and suffering.

But crap is also an acronym. An acronym that I created that stands for **C**ondition **R**esponses **A**utomatic **P**rogramming.

It is how the energetic connections of our neurons are fired and wired within our brains. It is the 98% of our unconscious programming that keeps us in cycles and loops. It is the triggers. It is our thoughts, our feelings, that create our experiences.

All of these physical and energetic connections are deeply connected to the biochemistry of our bodies, the neuroplasticity of our brains, the electromagnetic connections between our heart and soul and the environment we live in, the electromagnetic connections of the Earth and the universe.

We are interconnected interrelated beings. We cannot be divided into the smallest common denominator the way we were taught with Newtonian physics. Part of the crap that we need to unlearn is that we are insignificant and don't matter. We must learn and truly understand how everything matters and everything is connected within and without us.

I always said that I wanted a life of stories. The old saying about being careful what you wish for is displayed here as I share my journey.

I am happy to say that when I share how I Unlearned my Crap it is not about venting or trauma sharing but instead to show the correlation of cause and effect in how our C.R.A.P. (Conditioned Responses Automatic Programming) are created.

I aim to shed light on the toxicity of our beliefs and the trauma caused to the body in the form of disease, mental health and stress/burnout.

My hope is that my Unlearning my Crap, my connecting the dots of cause and effect will shed light on your own journey to Unlearn the Crap that is disempowering you.

I believe that we are in a pivotal moment of time, where the speed of evolution and the breakdown of our unsustainable systems are coinciding with the rise of individual empowerment. I believe that we are moving from the minority holding the control, power and wealth while the majority are feeding their greed through being kept as consumers and workers, indentured servants through debt and pay checks, to the system being reversed.

I believe that each of us has a unique contribution and the world is waiting for us to empower ourselves. We all have a purpose and a mission. When we identify and learn to live our lives in service to that purpose and mission, we create our peace, passion and prosperity.

I believe that the call has never been stronger for collaboration and cooperation. I believe that when we all live in our truest self, aligned in our body, mind and soul, that we can solve all the world's problems.

I don't believe that there is nothing we can't solve, no environmental problem, no hunger problem, no war, no hatred or prejudice if we use our true human gifts of compassion, imagination, creativity, love and problem solving.

My contribution is using my own journey, my own learnings to shed light and help my clients identify and quickly Unlearn the Crap that is holding them back. I am creating a collaborative community where we share our unique gifts and ask for what we need. I am working with my clients individually and collectively.

That is my purpose. My voice. My gift.

What is yours?

What is in your way? What CRAP do you need to Unlearn? What gifts are you not sharing because there is crap in your way?

I hope that by reading this book, I not only help you identify with your growth areas, but also help you clear your roadblocks to help you live your true mission and purpose with freedom.

INTRODUCTION

He almost killed me.

He said he tried.

I get that it wasn't his fault. NOW. He had his own Crap to Unlearn, but, in the meantime, it left me with my literal life-or-death choice.

I chose Life.

That was the beginning of Unlearn the Crap and the precise moment my life forever changed.

We all have pivotal moments where life alters into a direction that is sudden and a complete trajectory change. Where nothing can or ever will be the same as it was before. Sometimes we think the changes are better. Sometimes we feel they are worse at the moment.

Thankfully, I have come to realize that, in the end, change is ALWAYS for the better.

This is My Unlearning the Crap Story.

I remember bits and pieces of that moment.

I remember maybe 2 or 3 police officers dragging me out of my bathtub. I was fully dressed; the water was running, and I had a knife.

I remember lying on a gurney being wheeled out of my home, while I sobbed, "Please don't do this. This is not what I want."

I remember waking up in the hospital with a security guard watching me and being totally out of my mind.

The rest of the pieces of my memory came later, and I am not sure if I remember it all, but let me start at the beginning of that day.

* * * *

That day began with my being so excited and happy. I had an appointment with the psychiatrist that afternoon, and I had such high expectations that I was finally going to have someone "fix" me.

I had been waiting for months to see this doctor. Because like Humpty Dumpty, I was broken into a million pieces and I had been struggling for so long. I was tired of being broken. I was tired of living in a constant state of devastation and defeat.

I still couldn't understand how this happened to ME. I was the strong one. I was the one who fixed everything for everyone. I was educated. I was successful. Breaking happened to other people, not to me.

So, how in the hell did I BREAK?

I anxiously waited to be called into his office. His office was in the hospital. He was the one who called me from the waiting room to go inside. I thought we were off to an amazing start with that fact. The actual Doctor was the one to bring me into his office.

That had to be a good sign. Right?

With all the trust in him, in the system, I sat across from this man and answered all his questions. He asked about every single trauma, stress, pain, and history of my life from childhood to today. I shared the sexual assaults. I shared the verbal and emotional abuse. I shared my normal upbringing. I shared how I tried to drown myself at 12 in our pool. I shared how I was a cutter as a teenager. I shared the never-ending stress that led to over 30 years of undiagnosed disease and pain in my body.

Without hesitation, I opened every wound allowing myself to be raw and vulnerable.

After all, he was my new doctor, and he was going to save me.

I trusted him. I trusted the medical system.

I trusted.

So, when he finished with his questions, and I was exhausted and drained after sharing an entire lifetime of pain, I can not even begin to share how shocked I was that his response to hearing everything was...

Here is your prescription. I will see you in a few months.

And I was dismissed. Brushed off. Sent away. Rejected. Abandoned.

AGAIN.

I drove away with the prescriptions in my hand and headed to my drug store and pharmacist. This pharmacist had been filling a concoction of drugs and meds for me for a while as I was spiraling. He knew I was struggling. I had been a science experiment for years.

But I knew something was very wrong. I could feel myself unwinding, spiraling down, down, down, like a funnel inside. The tears streamed down my face silently.

I sat in the pharmacy chair waiting for my pills, face soaking wet, isolated, and alone.

And I sensed that I was in big trouble. I could feel myself losing control of myself.

I called out to friends to see if they wanted a visit. I knew it was a workday for most people, and I did not want to be a burden, so I accepted it when they were busy living their lives. They had no idea what state I was in, and we didn't connect.

I reached out to my family. They were busy.

My last call in the car, driving home with new pills, was to my ex. We had just broken up. He was part of the "everything that I lost" when I lost it all – my money, my home, my health, my relationship, my family, and my friends.

I blamed him.

He was going through his own kind of hell, and his ugly- hit my ugly, and we created a huge mess together. I can say that now, but at the time, all I could see was his ugly and that his ugly did this **TO ME**.

And I was fucking angry.

I spewed all my anger at him. Maybe anger would keep me from totally spiraling out of control. I had no idea. I just knew that I was not in a good place, and I wasn't safe to be alone. Plus, it felt good to dump all of this on HIM.

He asked if I wanted him to come over. I said yes, but he had to know and be able to handle the fact that I was not doing well. My ex liked to live in a place of "good and easy" . He didn't like to dredge up the past or face messy emotions. I was the Queen of Suppression and he was the King of Avoidance.

There was nothing that I could do or say that would make it easy for him if he chose to be there for me. There was no mask or fantasy that would make him coming over to my new place a happy social visit.

Knowing this, he thought it might be best to wait for another day.

And there it was. My truth.

I was alone.

Nobody was coming to save me. Not my family. Not my friends. Not the doctors. Not the system.

And not him, either.

Once home, I threw my phone across the room in anger, desperation, and total frustration.

I went to the kitchen. I sharpened the knife.

I went to the bathroom and got in the tub, fully dressed. I didn't want to leave a mess for anyone to clean up. I didn't want a stranger to find me naked. I had enough body shame already, I wasn't going to allow that final indignity.

I ran the bath water but didn't put the plug in.

I remember sobbing so hard that I couldn't catch my breath. I remember the sounds coming out of me didn't sound human. I remember feeling detached and disconnected from my physical body. Disconnected from my heart. Disconnected from myself. Disconnected from life.

And I felt relief with the disconnection.

I remember rubbing the knife on my wrists, and I remember the feeling of sweet relief, a feeling I remembered well from my teenage years when I would cut my arms in order to release the pain from the inside. The sharpness of the knife was familiar and actually comforting. I found myself savouring that feeling, the pleasure of the pain. There my pain was being replaced with relief. It was comforting.

And then, I was being roughly dragged out of my tub.

It was all so confusing. I was locked in my apartment. I was alone. I had closed the bedroom door to keep my cat safe and away from me. I had closed the bathroom door.

Where did these police officers come from? Why were they in my home, my bathroom? Why were they forcing me onto a gurney and dragging me to the hospital against my will?

I don't remember getting into the ambulance. I don't remember the drive there. I don't remember being checked into an emergency room.

I DO remember waking up so depressed that I was there, and I had failed. I had even failed at this.

I DO remember being empty in my mind and spirit. I DO remember feeling disconnected and disassociated from who I thought I was. I DO remember just lying there, staring out into space.

I remember them telling me that I was being "formed," and that meant I was being held against my will. I remember feeling so out of control of my own self and my own life.

And then...

Like a stranger emerging from a night fog, I felt myself returning.

Slowly...

I could feel my mind coming back to me.

Piece by piece...

Moment by moment...

It was the most amazing sensation, like connecting with a long, lost friend.

I was back.

Almost 24 hours after I left that psychiatrist's office, my brain and sanity came back to me.

I told the nurses that I was okay now.

They called in the attending psychiatrist to evaluate me. I told him about my appointment with his colleague, in this very hospital. I told him about the last 6 months, about how I had lost everything. I told him about the last year that I had just endured, sexual abuse by a supposed girl "friend", verbal and emotional abuse by an employer, the hell that my relationship had become. I told him about my physical illnesses with fibromyalgia, about constant never-ending pain all over my body, about my osteoarthritis, and about my adrenal fatigue. I told him about the loss of my extended family after the passing of my parents 7 weeks apart. I told him about my failed marriage, I told him about the addictions in my circles, the traumas, the abuses. I told him everything. I told him everything that I had just shared with the doctor yesterday.

And his response was **AMAZING**.

He told me that it made perfect sense why I found myself in the emergency room of the hospital. He empathized that I had endured more than I could handle, and that made perfect sense to him.

Everyone has a breaking point, and I had hit mine. I was broken. But I was sane again as well.

He believed me when I said I was fine, and he should have because I really was fine again. I was cognitively aware of my situation, and I knew my life was in my hands.

He released me and wished me well.

This experience was the first step to my self-healing. And then, another pivotal event occurred, and that forever changed the trajectory of my life.

* * * *

When I returned to the original psychiatrist's office, and I shared with him what happened after I saw him last, his response was also AMAZING, but not in the good way that I had just experienced in that emergency room.

He said words that I will never forget.

He said words that forever changed me and the trajectory of my life.

He said his role in my healing was **ONLY** to ensure that I was adequately medicated. His role was **ONLY** in the drugs he prescribed. His role was **NOT** in healing me.

I realized that if I was going to heal, the healing had to come **FROM ME**.

Nobody was going to save me. Nobody was putting Humpty Dumpty back together again.

If it was to be,
It was up to me.

I am 15 years old, and I have skipped school in order to stay home and clean the house. I am on my hands and knees and scrubbing the floor with a toothbrush to ensure that not one spec of dirt remains.

The music is blaring so loud, and I am wailing along at the top of my lungs with silent tears flowing down my face. The song is from The Gatlin Brothers, and it is called "Broken Lady."

I am the Broken Lady, even though I am still a child.

In my mind, if I create the perfect environment, then I will live a happy life. My parent's stress has become my responsibility. My sister is my responsibility. Everything is up to me. Where did this come from?

I was never told that. It was never inferred. Yet it was a part of my bodily structure, my thoughts, my beliefs, and my actions.

Broken Lady - Lyrics by Larry Gatlin

She's a broken lady
Waiting to be mended
Like a potter would mend
A broken vase
A broken lady
Waiting to be mended
And have what's left of the pieces
Put back in place
Her love is like a fortress
Around a man she would have died for
Taking care, to take care of all he needed
But the lady's fortress slowly turned into a prison
And the warning signs he gave, she never heeded
She vowed every morning
That what God joined together
No one else in the world could pull apart
Then the walls came tumbling to the ground
And her world came crashing down around her heart
Her heart
Now she's a broken lady
Waiting to be mended
Like a potter would mend
A broken vase
A broken lady
Waiting to be mended
And have what's left of the pieces
Put back in place
She's a broken lady
Waiting to be mended
And have what's left of the pieces
Put back in place

My First Reality

When I think about my childhood, all I can remember is being happy.

I now know the root of my issues are trauma-based, and most result from childhood, so if what I remember is happy times, where did my trauma come from?

I think everything changed when I was around 12. It was about that time that I experienced what I call major and minor traumas that, in hindsight, I can see had a profound effect on me.

The first was when I got my period. I knew I would be getting it soon. We had just finished having "health" classes that talked about the basic reproductive cycle and that it happened. That was all that I really knew. It was never talked about in my home, not puberty, not sex, not our reproductive cycle, or basically anything about the body.

As a latchkey kid, it was up to me to get up and get ready for school and make sure that I was there on time. Both of my parents were working and left for work before I got up. So, when I went to the bathroom that morning and found blood, I froze. I had no idea what to do or how to handle it so I did what any other normal person would do, I ignored it.

I got dressed and headed to school like everything was normal, and I truly tried to believe it was. But I was getting wetter and wetter. Thank God, lunch came soon, and it was then that I ran like a world-class sprinter home. I called my mom at work, which was not something that I was supposed to do unless it was really important. I deemed this important because I had no idea how to handle what was happening.

"Mom," I said, "I think I got my period."

In my mother's typical style, her response was, "What do you mean you think?"

"Okay, okay," I told her, "I got my period."

Then, my mother lowered her voice into a whisper on the phone and told me where to find the feminine products and what to do with them. It was the mid-70s, and when you hear that saying 'you've come a long way, Baby', I truly always think of feminine products.

I used my first pad that day, returning to school in different clothes than I arrived that morning, feeling like my legs had a large pillow between them, walking with an unusual gait because of this intrusion. I tried to pretend everything was normal. But nothing felt normal. I felt like I had a neon sign, and everyone knew.

My period was something to be celebrated by my grandmother.

I had just become a woman, according to her. My grandmother convinced my dad to let me get my ears pierced to celebrate this milestone. Based on everything that my father felt was "proper" for a girl to do, earrings were not one of them. But he caved in. He was the lone-wolf male of our household, and he couldn't fight every battle against the feminine in the house. His only condition was that I never wear hoop earrings. Only bad girls did that.

My grandmother worked in a hair salon in the local mall, and that was where the deed was to happen. The gun that they used to put the first earring in felt like a bullet going through me—as if I knew what a bullet should feel like. But it hurt. It hurt badly. I almost didn't get the second ear done because it hurt so bad, but that was the first time I remember 'sucking it up, buttercup' and doing what was expected of me, regardless of how much it hurt.

When it was done, I ran. I ran through the mall, trying to get the breeze of the air rushing along my ears to alleviate the burning sensation.

So, even though I didn't ask for my period or the pierced ears, now I was different, and so was my ideal life.

* * * *

One day, I was walking home from the local mall with my best friend and her baby sister. We cut through the schoolyard to get home. I didn't know how not to feel safe, this was my school, my neighborhood, and it was the middle of the day.

So, when 5 boys came out of nowhere and attacked me, I was shocked and paralyzed. They told me what they were going to do. They told me they were going to rape me. They used those words. Four of the boys each grabbed a limb to hold me down, while the fifth one was wrestling with my pants to get them off.

I looked over at my friend, who was there with her baby sister, and I screamed to get her out of there, don't let her see this. So, my friend did just that, she ran with her sister to shield her from this torment.

Then, with them safely out of watch, the strength of a lion came over me, and I wrestled, squirmed, and fought back. I got one leg free and used it to kick the boy who was trying to get my pants off me in the nuts so hard that he rolled off me. With that much leverage and anger surging through my veins, I was able to break free from the last 3 boys trying to contain me so that they could have their fun.

And I ran again.

Only this time, I wasn't running to feel the air brush softly past my burning ears. This time I was running with surging fear and, I guess, pure adrenaline. When we got safely away, and we were close to my home, my father drove past us. I ignored him and walked past my house to get to my friend's home.

I couldn't let my father see me or know what happened, after all, I deserved what I got. I was wearing the forbidden hoop earrings, and I needed to get them off before I could face my parents.

I went to my best friend's home, removed the evidence of my wantonness, and told my friend's mother what had happened. She was the first person to console me and comfort me. When I felt composed enough, I walked back home and told my parents what happened.

But what really affected me about that day was my mother's response. "Why, Kathy, did you tell your friend's mother first? Why didn't you come to us?"

Here I was dealing with a major trauma and desperately needing her to comfort me. I was scared. I was in new dangerous, unsafe waters that I didn't know how to handle. Yet, my focus became about her feelings and the guilt that she was feeling badly.

I couldn't answer her. How could I admit it was my fault, I had broken the cardinal rule of wearing those damn hoop earrings. My parents never ever knew the truth that I took responsibility and felt it was my fault because I was wearing hoop earrings. My parents died and we NEVER discussed this incident again.

They immediately called the police, and I had to recount the incident and look through books and books of mugshots, trying to find the faces of the boys who attacked me. That process went on for months.

I never saw his face in those books. But when I saw his face about 10 years later, I immediately KNEW it was HIM, and the terror came flooding back into my body, and so did the freeze. I just stared at him.

And I did nothing. I said nothing.

I already had a pattern of freezing established, and it would take a lifetime to break. The pattern of other's feelings were more important than mine was tied into my belief system.

* * * *

As young girls trying to be 'cool', we used to take our jeans and put them on inside out. Then we could pin the pants so that they were literally skin-tight and sew them to our exact shape. I was a lousy seamstress at age 12, so I think I reinforced those stitches by sewing over the top of each row. Nothing was going to have those seams break open on me.

The problem became in putting them back on. That required lying down on the bed, using a coat hanger looped into the zipper, and then, by the magic of leverage, zipping up those pants. Going to the bathroom to repeat this was absolutely out of the question, but I looked good.

This became my new go-to outfit. I strutted and felt good. My body was beginning to develop, I was one of the first in my group to develop 'buds', and it felt fun and alive.

That year my parents took us to Florida for Christmas break. I was a 12-year-old, and I was wearing an orange string bikini (funny how string bikini was ok, but hoop earrings were not).

I was splashing in the waves of the ocean and having so much fun, and I guess so were the waves. Without my knowing it, the strings loosened, and my top came off and was swallowed up by the waves. Jumping up and down in the waves, I was now, for a brief moment, showing my new buds off to the world.

Now, we were off to the local mall and my mom bought me my first bra. So much for those buds being fun. Now they had to be hidden and locked up. I believe that was my first experience with shame.

On the last day of school that year, we had an assembly outside in the schoolyard. I was wearing a tube top dress that had spaghetti straps. One of the straps had broken during the day, so I had tucked it in and so the dress was now strapless. One of the boys, who was my friend, hooked his finger into my dress top and did a tug. My dress came flying down around my knees, and I stood there all in the glory for the school to see me. I never did have those horrible nightmares of finding myself naked in public because I had lived it. I knew the shame, the embarrassment, the true pure vulnerability of being exposed by someone I trusted.

* * * *

One day, I was doing my paper route on a Saturday morning. I loved to deliver the Saturday paper on my wagon because I could collect enough money on the route to buy myself a treat. Halfway through my route, at the point that I had to do a UTurn and reverse down the other side of the street, was an Italian bakery. There, I discovered the joy of the cannoli.

Every Saturday, I made sure that I collected just enough money so that I could indulge in my secret treat, and this one particular day was no different.

I woke up and put my papers together because they came in sections, and the Saturday paper had so many components. I had to insert the lifestyle section, where the comics lived during the week, but on weekends, it was special, and they were separate and came in color. I had to insert the weekly TV guide so we knew what to watch, and when it came on, so we could plan our week around the TV schedule.

I loaded everything up in my cart and began my route. At the halfway point, I stopped and got my weekly treat and savored every morsel. God, I loved food. I loved the texture, the way it made my mouth come alive, and how happy it made me feel.

After my indulgence, I would complete my route and enjoy the rest of my Saturday. I usually ended the route by stopping at my friend's house, maybe having lunch with her family or hanging out with my other friends. During those days, I could go out and do whatever I wanted, and go wherever I wanted, I just needed to be home before the streetlights came on.

But this Saturday was going to be different, and I had no warning.

I think it was mid-afternoon when I arrived home, with my wagon in tow, wearing my newfound tight jeans and the obligatory new bra. My tummy was happy, and so was I.

But my mother was not. She was furious. She met me in the driveway, demanding to know where I had been. I was so surprised because this was what I did every Saturday morning. Why was she so mad at me?

It appeared that her cousins and family had arrived, and they had been waiting for me. In hindsight, I am sure my mother was embarrassed that she couldn't answer their questions about my whereabouts and when I would be home, and to this day, I do not remember ever being told that I needed to finish my paper route routine any earlier than normal, but, obviously, my mother had a different version of those events.

She was angry and mortified at my attire. She looked me up and down, slapped me in the face, and called me a slut. She told me to go into the house, change my clothes, and then, when I was looking respectful, join them in the backyard with her cousins, the perfect family.

We lived in a semi-detached home on a cul-de-sac, or court as we called it. I loved that place so much. We had a pool in the backyard, which was very unusual for the neighborhood, so we were the center of the gathering. Our entire social lives centered around our house for all members of the family. In the summer, we swam in the pool, and it's where my girlfriends and I skinny dipped for the first time. In the winter, we could toboggan on the hill in the center of the court that was created by the snowplow because we used to get a lot of snow.

I had a large group of friends, and we called ourselves the gang. Some of the gang were boys older than me, but that was okay because my dad loved having the boys over. They were the sons he always wanted, and when they were around, he could do boy things with them. Our gang was large, and we were fierce, and we were envied because of how close we all were to each other.

Because my parents worked so hard and we came home from school long before they arrived, it made perfect sense to my parents that it became our responsibility to make sure that the house was clean before they came home. I would enlist the help of my gang to clean the house. We had a long shag carpet that needed to be raked after it was vacuumed. Once that was done, every single footstep became like footsteps in the sand, the pristine perfection of it was gone until the next day when the process repeated.

We needed to put all the shoes away from the front hall, make sure the dishes were washed and put away, and the house dusted. Each of my friends knew their specific role and would help us clean up so we could go out and play.

But of course, this was my responsibility, and not every day did my friends want to clean someone else's house. Sometimes, they just wanted to play. I did too, so I couldn't blame them.

If I did not do the daily cleaning, I would come home to my mother saying, "All I ask for is that I come home to a clean house after a long day at work. Is that too much to ask for?" That question is still a massive trigger for me today. Like if someone thinks it's a small thing to ask for, then I should be required to obey.

So, I took it on. It was my responsibility to make sure that my parents came home from work happy.

Another pattern was set. What people needed and wanted and how they needed and wanted it, was my responsibility, and if they were unhappy with how I did it, it was my fault.

One day, I remember coming home from school, and I was overwhelmed and had no idea how to handle it. I went out in the backyard to the happy place of the pool and decided to try and drown myself.

I jumped in the pool, held my breath, and tried to leave my problems behind. Little did I know that it is almost impossible to drown yourself because your body will force you to breathe even if you try to override it. Your body will take care of itself if you don't listen. Another life lesson that would take me a lifetime to appreciate and truly honor.

When my mother came home, I told her what I had tried to do. In her young, exasperated, exhausted place, her response was, "That would be a fine thing to come home and find after a long hard day at work."

I had failed again. I had failed to find solace for what I was feeling, and I had failed to please my mother again.

I don't remember ever being told about how I was conceived and how she became a teenage underage bride. It feels like I always knew it. My mother carried her shame and her duty and did her best to not glamorize her success. She wanted to make sure that I did not repeat her mistake by following in her path. In her way, she was trying to protect me, trying to have me live up to my personal potential, but all I heard was I was not wanted or planned. All it meant to me was I had ruined my mother's life, and I did not belong. I carried around a burden of constantly wanting to please everyone. It was never a conscious thought process. It was just an underlying fact like breathing. It just was, and I had accepted this unconscious belief as my truth and fate in life.

I really want to make sure that I do not paint my mother as a bad person or a bad mother. She was young, beautiful, and my hero. I loved and adored her. She was everything I wanted to grow up to be. She was doing the best she could every single day, but she was not trained or prepared for how her life evolved, how to be a mother of a 12-year-old when she was only 28 herself.

She had no idea how the brain worked, how beliefs were created, and how our DNA gets wired by our environment. She didn't know about the central nervous system and suppressed emotions.

Nobody did.

So, she had absolutely no idea how those small things she said and did affected me. I know that if she did, she would have moved heaven and earth to do things differently. She loved me dearly. But she had her own Crap to Unlearn. And after all, they were just words, what lasting harm could words actually do?

Yes, age 12 changed everything for me and about me. I would never be the same happy naive child again. Everything would now become so freaking hard.

My World Changed

Growing up for me was a stark contrast to each stage of my life. In my early years, I was extremely social. I was actually the center, the glue of our "gang". Everyone met at my house, everyone hung out at my place. My parents were the cool ones, and we had a pool.

My group were fierce protectors of each other, and we did everything together. The majority of the boys were about 2 years older than me, and my father loved it. My dad was the only testosterone in our home; he joked that even the pets were female. I know he felt isolated at times and like it was him against us. The boys coming around really helped.

My dad was a hobby drag racer and spent his weekends tinkering with his car. He had a Hemi Orange Duster that he dragged at the local race track, and he was pretty good at it. He won a few trophies and got published in the local paper once as well.

My dad was also a fierce learner, and anything that needed to be done, he learned how to do it. He did all the home improvements, from building fireplaces and fences to electrical, plumbing, you name it.

My dad's shop was in the basement, and the door was lined inside with Playboy centerfolds. My dad loved women, their beauty, and their curves, and my mom was his perfect playmate. The boys loved going to hang out in the basement, and they always commented on how sexy my mom was. She was only 16 years older than me, and when she drove up in that Hemi Orange Duster that we could hear a mile away and slung her long legs out of the car... well, the boys loved watching her. I wonder if my gang loved my parents more than me as I write this. But it doesn't matter, either way, they were my family, my tribe, my community, and I loved every single one of them.

We were the X Generation, and we had free rein to run and explore, as long as we were home before the streetlights came on.

My father had a Ford van that he had decked out for us to travel and go camping in. It was 2-toned, brown, and the inside was orange fluffy fabric for the bench seats that turned into a bed. The back door had a sticker that said, "If this van's rockin', don't bother knockin'". I thought that meant the music was being played loud to leave us alone. I was so naive.

We used to take that van and travel across the USA and Canada. My parents would sleep inside the van on the convertible bed and my sister and I would sleep outside in a tent. When it wasn't converted into a bed, the van had a table with bench seating. We could sit there, play games, look at the window, make and eat food. Between the table and the driver's seat we had all that we needed for food and drinks, so we could travel and still meet (MOST) of our needs.

In one of those trips, I guess I didn't manage my intake very well and didn't understand the universal law of cause and effect, because eventually what goes in must come out. I told my dad that I needed to go to the bathroom. He said we could stop when we ran out of gas and needed to refuel and told me to hold it.

As my desperation grew, I watched that fuel gauge with so much intensity, wishing for it to hit empty as soon as possible. Just as it neared empty and I thought to myself, ok I can hold on to my bladder now, my relief time is near, my father reached down and hit a switch. He had dual gas tanks which meant that when one was empty he could just flip the switch and the gauge would return to full and we could continue driving.

I was mortified and told him that I couldn't hold on any longer. We needed to stop now. I was told to hang on, we were almost at our camping spot and I could go then.

Almost there obviously had different meanings for him and me. I was in so much pain and felt like I was going to explode and almost meant another couple of hours.

But then we arrived at the camping site and as we were entering, I saw the public bathrooms and begged him to please stop and let me out, but it was almost dark and he wanted to find the location first. He said I could go back as soon as we found our spot.

When we arrived at our spot and the vehicle finally stopped, I ripped open that sliding door with so much force and ran as fast as I could. My sister was with me and she knew how badly I had to go so she became very confused when I just stopped running and began to cry.

My body had passed its limits. The running was too much for my bladder to handle, and my body took care of my desperation without any regard to the humiliation that would follow.

I slowly walked back with my head hung low and crying. I was a young teen and my jeans were soaked with urine. I had failed and everyone could see it.

My mother used to brag that she was so perfect that she didn't have bodily functions. I just proved to everyone that I was so far from perfect, that not only did I have them, but I couldn't control them.

Learning to control my body, suppress my needs, reduce the amount of fluid I let into my body were going to be major recurring themes for me that I would pay dearly for.

* * * *

My grandfather (my dad's dad) was extremely entrepreneurial and very forward-thinking. He was a major player in our area, bringing CB radios to the car users, and my dad loved his. It hung from the roof of the van, and we had "handles." My dad, of course, was "The Captain", and my mom was "The Crew." My CB handle was "The Sleeper" because I could really really sleep deep, and it was impossible to wake me up.

My father figured out that if he installed a 2-way switch and put a speaker under the hood of the van, he could turn his CB radio into a loudspeaker, which he used on drivers who were not obeying The Captain's rules of the road (so embarrassing) and, for me, he could use it to drive around the neighborhood and call my full name over the speaker.

"Kaaa-thh-ee Baall-dwinnn, it's time to come home. Where are you?"

My gang friends just loved that. They thought it was hilarious, and I would be chased down in the neighborhood, "Kathy, the van is on the lookout for you." I was so embarrassed that I would hide from it and find my own way home independent of the free ride. No way was I going to let my father know that his torture was working.

My mother, on the other hand, thought it was crude to yell my name out the door, calling for me to come home. So, she thought it was "classy" to ring a bell. She bought a bell that one might have used for the butler or maid in high-class societies (we were not). We lived in a semi-detached house in a middle-class neighborhood. When it was time for me to come home, she would step outside on the front porch and ring the bell.

Ring, Ring, Ring, Ring.

Again, I would hide. It might as well have been a cowbell, as far as I was concerned. My friends loved it and taunted me with the bell as much as they did with the bullhorn.

That was also the signal to my friends that after dinner, they were always welcome to come hang out and watch TV with the family. We had a long wooden TV console unit, and the TV was a part of it, which meant that the best seat was lying down on the floor. My friends would gather around, and we would watch Mork and Mindy, or whatever other show was on.

It wasn't just my parents that were cool back then, either. One of my dear friends' parents would invite me over to play euchre with them on a Saturday night. We would play and listen to Meat Loaf's "Bat Out of Hell" record playing on the record player. Even though I was only in grade 8, sitting there at the table with the adults, feeling like we were all friends, was such an important lesson for me. It was a lesson that both served me and led me astray in the future. Everything in my life was full of contradictions.

My best friend's family became my family as well. I would hang out with them and go visit them independently of my friends, and I could trust and feel totally comfortable with them. My parents were controlling, so in my best friend's home I could just be me: I could hang out with boys, I could smoke, but I also had to do chores and be a part of their household routines. If you could adapt to the household, you were welcomed. I loved being able to be free to be me, and I spent a lot of time there.

Everything was easy, fun, and comfortable for me. I had friends, I had a support system, I had neighborhood and community.

I could be free and be safe.

But the 70s were times of excess and wanting more, and my parents had achieved their best life in that neighborhood. I was graduating from grade school and about to enter high school. The local high school was where my gang already were attending, so I was thrilled to be joining them there, but it was also known as the local drug school.

One of the neighbors on our street was a cop, and I guess he warned my parents about the school because the next thing I knew, my parents had bought a new house, and we were moving across town. It might as well have been to a totally different country for me. We moved in the middle of the last year of grade school, and my life forever changed.

My parents were trying to ensure that I had the best life possible and so they thought they were doing the correct thing moving us across town. The high school that I was going to just had a school shooting about 2 years before. School shootings were never heard of when I was growing up especially in Canada where nobody had guns that we were aware of. My mother worked with the shooter's father, and she was well aware that this young man was very troubled. She saw this as an isolated incident of a poor young man struggling, even though he came from a "good" family.

I saw it as doom and gloom, and it was an omen of how my life would evolve.

The gang helped us get the house ready before we moved in. They all came, and we had a painting party in the basement to seal the concrete. They had their own cars, so they drove back and forth. I was too young to drive, so I was at their mercy as to when we saw each other, but that painting party was so much fun. There was probably more paint on us than there was on the floor, but we laughed. I hoped that the move to this beautiful brand new house could come with my friends, and maybe it wouldn't be so bad.

So, with the naivete of a young girl who had a safe and happy life, I moved and entered my new school. Day 1 proved to me that I was not in Kansas anymore. The cool girls, the mean girls, decided that they did not like a new girl, and they did not like me. They ganged up on me, they called me names, and they deemed me a "slut". I was given the nickname of 'boobs' because those damn buds had kept growing.

They created rumors about me that stayed with me through my entire high school years. They did it because they could, I guess. After all, I had just arrived at the school, I didn't know a soul, and yet this new label was attached to me.

I had just entered a war zone where I would not fit in, and I did not belong. The only safety I had were the boys and my writing. The boys hung out with me, and we had fun, like running and splashing in the puddles of the rain, or roughhousing. They were not trying to hit on me, and actually, I was seen as their sister and friend and never romantically. With the boys, I could laugh, play, and be myself. With the girls, I had to hide and protect myself.

And when the pain came, which it always did, I would hide at recess and write poetry. It just poured out of me. All the isolation, loneliness, missing having friends, being accepted and belonging, all came out in my poetry.

I carried those poems with me for most of my adult life. Unfortunately they were lost at the same time as I lost my parents.

I wrote a poem about what it was like to be elderly and have Alzheimer's which my teacher loved. I remember her saying how rare it was for someone so young to have such empathy and insight into an experience that I had no knowledge of. The poem began with each line of " I remember..." Even after all these years I still remember the last lines...

"But they don't remember that I remember."

Some of my other poems were deep passionate love letters to the love I dreamt of having. They were filled with longing, pain and passion.

Some of the poems were to purge out the constant pain I carried deep in my soul, the loneliness, the unworthiness and longing for meaning.

I was alone and a misfit in high school. I was smart but not smart enough to be with the "brainers". I didn't party or do drugs so I didn't fit in with the "stoners." I was not athletic so I definitely didn't fit with the "jocks." There was no place that I fit.

And that school shooting haunted me. When I walked around that high school, I could always feel the presence of the screams of terror and hear the bullets flying when I walked in the corridor just outside of the counselor's office. I could viscerally feel it and sometimes I felt like I could see the blood on the locker doors or the bullet holes penetrating them. I clearly remember hearing about John Lennon's death at the exact spot that the shooter had killed his victims.

It was almost as if that shooting by that poor tortured boy paved the way for my own experience.

* * * *

The funny thing is that for my parents, this move was the best thing for their social life. The street we moved to was all people like my parents, around their age and they all blended like it was planned. The street became my parents' gang, and they had a social life that I envied and missed.

The neighbours all bonded and became lifelong friends. Their social life was filled with constant parties and my mother was the perfect hostess. I absolutely loved her creativity when it came to entertaining. I remember one party was a going away party for a neighbour who was moving away. The couple that had sold their house were having dinner across the street. While the dinner party was going on, everyone got to work.

Across the street at their home, their front yard was decorated like a dilapidated graveyard and if you read the inscriptions on each cross, each had an inside joke about memories of their living there.

When it came time for dessert, the entire neighbourhood came into the dinner party dressed as a Mardi Gras parade, with music playing and wailing at the loss of loved ones. The hosts of the party got up and joined the procession as if their guests were not even there any longer. It was played like they were invisible and had no idea what was going on, other than to follow along where the party / funeral ended at our house with a full on wake.

The piece de resistance of the wake was when one of the neighbours got up to read their eulogy and read from one of their children's story books. It had no significance other than being totally nonsensical.

My parents hosted annual lobsterfest parties where we cooked dozens of lobsters over an open flame bbq in the backyard in a large drum. Everyone would eat their messy lobster at the picnic table and then jump in the pool to wash off.

There was always a party or an event. They were a tight group of friends and they opened their arms to others joining in. There was dancing until the wee hours of the morning. There were multi course dinners that rivalled Michelin star dining. There were impromptu get-togethers that would build lifelong memories.

To this day, I long for my gang – my vibrant, safe social life that I had as a child, and my parents created in their best years. I long to create the safety of that community. It is probably one of the driving forces behind my serving my clients and community today.

* * * *

Our next door neighbors in the new house were our family friends. We did so much together and I have some amazing memories of both of them. The wife and I would dance together to songs that still make me smile. She helped me get some of my first jobs. She was beautiful, successful and a total role model for me.

Her husband was a charmer. He had a very risky job and obviously loved the adrenaline rushes. He took a personal liking to me and in hindsight

I can see how he was grooming me. But at the time, a girl who had lost her tribe, who was rejected by her peers, who was an outsider, his attention filled a deep need in me.

And it was confusing.

I knew it was wrong but yet I craved it. I adored his wife and felt guilty by his attention. He never abused me but he crossed and danced on the line. He would sit too close. He would have his hand just close enough to mine to feel the electricity. He would wink secret winks at me. When we went to the amusement park as a group, he would take me on rides alone, hold my hand, put his arm around me and we would laugh at the looks that people gave us. I think he relished the brazen way he strutted around as a 40 something man with a teenage girl, knowing that he could feign innocence if ever confronted.

He would tell me that when I turned 21 he was coming to take me on a date. He told me that so often that I actually expected him to turn up when I was 21 even though he had moved away long before then as he moved on to his next conquest while having an affair on his wife.

Unfortunately, I was to have this experience repeated numerous times with family friends, executives at work, and socially. One family friend offered me an unlimited credit card if I would have sex with him. A manager at work created a cassette tape of love songs that he said he thought of me when he heard them. Another Executive asked if I would go to his car with him and remove my top so he could play with my breasts. He assured me he didn't want to have an affair, he just wanted to touch me. I wish the list of stories like these ended here, but there are so many more that I endured. It just kept happening over and over again which just eroded my self worth. The message that I was getting was my value resided in people using and abusing me with zero regard for me as a person.

Pleasure and needs were always in conflict and I didn't have a clear understanding of any of it.

If only I had been taught about boundaries and finding my own self worth, then I would not have become easy prey to be used and abused. I now know that my internal beliefs energetically brought the worst to me. Knowing what I know about energy now, I would have been repelling the very things that I desperately sought after.

* * * *

My first job was at the mall. One of my parents' friends owned a clothing store in the mall, and I was given the opportunity to work there and make some money. I loved it, and I was a natural. I could help women look at themselves in the mirror, and with honesty, tell them what made them look fantastic and what didn't. I had no problem with the truth because there was always an answer and a solution.

The mall had the obligatory food court where I would go and get my lunch or dinner. In the middle of the aisle, there was a donut shop and remembering the happy feelings of the Italian bakery of my childhood, I loved to go there. The front glass was angled so that you could see the variety of delicious goods and lean up on it comfortably.

One day, I was doing just that, I had placed my order for my treat and was talking to the server leaning on the counter. But something wasn't right. I felt someone leaning on me, you know that feeling when you are trapped in a crowd and someone else's body is touching yours, and it feels so uncomfortable, but you can't complain because everyone was in the same boat? Well, that was how I was feeling.

Until I could feel the person leaning on me begin to gyrate against my behind. That didn't make sense. I must be imagining it. I turned my head to see what was happening, and there was no big crowd pushing someone into me. It was just a single man. I was so confused and just didn't understand, but he had moved away, so I brushed it off and returned to my conversation with the server.

And then, he did it again. Only this time, the gyrating was pushing hard and fast on my bum, and I did not like it at all. I whipped my head around, and he took off.

What the hell was that?

When I returned to the store still in shock of what happened, the local security guard walked by. I called him over and laughingly told him what happened. I was still so naive that I did not get the severity of it. While I was telling him what happened, that man was walking behind a woman, gyrating against her WHILE she was walking. I was amazed actually at the talent it took to be in rhythm with how he was doing it, and I immediately pointed it out to the security guard—look, there he is and he is doing it to that woman.

The security guard took off and tried to catch him, but he got away.

Later that day, the guard returned with the police. It seemed that guy had been caught ejaculating on a display of women's panties in a store and had been arrested. I was asked to give my statement, which I did. Again, I was with the police having to give a statement and identify a sexual predator, only this time, I knew what he looked like, and they had him in custody.

That statement resulted in my having to go to court to testify. I remember being a young, terrified girl, sitting outside the local courtroom, waiting to go in and testify, all alone. In order to feel a little safer and secure, I remember using the pay phone on the wall to call my mom while she was at work again. She was always the one that I called when I needed comforting, and her words could always give me courage.

But yet, I was still there in a courtroom, facing the unknown, terrified and alone. I really was establishing a pattern of crap of beliefs.

I never did have to testify. The case was remanded for another day, and the second time I had to go to court for the trial, I was dismissed without testifying. They must have come up with a deal, but I was never told why after all this that I had gone through, I was dismissed and no longer needed to share my story. It just ended there without any fanfare. Just poof, move on. Put it behind you.

* * * *

I lost my virginity at the age of 16 and 1 month. I was the last of my friends to achieve this milestone, and it happened without my knowing it was going to happen or a conscious choice to have it happen.

I was in Florida, staying with my grandparents. They owned a home there, and I loved it. My grandfather had promised me a trip to Europe for my high school graduation, and I had made a trade with him, bringing my sister and me to Florida with them in exchange for the trip to Europe.

I am sure my grandparents were thrilled that we wanted to spend time with them and so they made it happen. When we arrived there, they had a neighbor named Patti, and she was a bit older than us, but she was so cool. Patti took us around and introduced us to her friends. Her friends were older and were into partying. I refused to do drugs, but I discovered a taste for alcohol that I liked. Everyone in my life drank, so it wasn't wrong of me to take shots of Jack Daniel's while playing a drinking game. It was one of those tongue-twister games that when you couldn't say the words, you needed to take a shot. I took a lot of shots, and I liked it.

I also discovered caffeine pills. If you took enough of those, you had such a fantastic feeling and so energized.

That was when I met him. Donny.

We went to Donny's house with his brother and Patti. Donny was 23, and I was 16. He stood at the foot of the driveway, working on his car, until he saw me. When he saw me, he stopped everything and didn't leave my side. I was in awe. This guy was HOT!!! What was he doing fawning all over me? But the attention of someone so gorgeous and so nice was irresistible.

I remember Donny invited me to dinner. We went to a seafood restaurant, and before the waitress came by, I excused myself and went to the bathroom. Here I was, playing adult, at 16 with a mouth full of braces, out on a date with the most gorgeous man I had ever seen. He looked like one of the movie stars that was popular on TV, and I was so awestruck that he was so interested in me that I was head over heels.

When I came back to the table, Donny told me that he had ordered me a Pina Colada. This would be my first one. The waitress came to bring the drinks and put them on the table, and she had a look of shock on her face. I knew what that meant. She knew I was way underage, and now she was serving an underage minor a drink with a gorgeous older man. I never ordered a second drink, knowing full well that she would have to deny me.

Donny and I hung out as much as possible. Then one day, I found myself alone with him at his house. Somehow everyone else went somewhere, and I just wanted to be wherever Donny was.

Our petting became heavy, and he wanted to make love to me. He actually used those words. They were the poetry and the love that I had been seeking. Here I was, 16, with a mouth full of braces, and this gorgeous man desired Me. It was too much to resist, and after all, I was pretty much an old maid by then, everyone I knew had already done it, so why shouldn't I?

Except, I was on my period. No, this would not work. Donny assured me that it did not bother him. He knew I was a virgin, and he was so kind, so gentle, so wonderful, and I was on those damn caffeine pills. The experience was euphoric for me. It was almost an out-of-body experience of pure pleasure. When it was over, Donny promised me round 2 soon.

Round 2 never ever happened. All our friends arrived back at his place, and I was so upset that I just started crying. I had just experienced heaven with an angel, and now it was over, and all I wanted was to go back.

Donny's brother asked me why I was crying. Donny was beside himself, beating himself up for upsetting me by taking my virginity. He had no idea how wrong he had it. I had no words to explain it, but I tried.

My only regret was that I was on my period.

I took an orange from Donny's tree with me and I carried that orange for over 25 years. It just petrified and became like a stone. But it was what I had at that moment and Donny, and I treasured it.

Donny begged me to stay in Florida with him. He wanted me to live with him, but I needed to go home, get those damn braces off and finish high school. I told him that was my plan and that I would be back.

We tried to stay in touch. We talked for hours into the night, a long distance from my home in Canada to Florida. We racked up hundreds of dollars in long-distance phone charges that my parents had to pay. My parents were furious, and they threatened to charge him with statutory rape. They threatened and tried to keep me away. They didn't know how to unhook the phone so I couldn't sneak it into my bedroom in the middle of the night to spend hours on the phone talking to him.

The fighting at home became too much for me, so I wrote Donny a letter telling him everything about how I felt. I told him about what that moment of losing my virginity meant to me, how much he meant to me, and how much I adored him. I promised to find him again when I was 18. I poured my heart and soul into that letter, and then I stopped calling him.

I put it in an envelope. I addressed it. I stamped it. I never put it in the mail. I found it years later. Donny obviously never knew why I just ghosted him. Years later, when I was 18 and returned to Florida, this time with my parents, I phoned Donny to see if we could meet and talk. He refused me. I can't blame him, after all, I just dumped him and broke his heart, and he had no idea why or what happened. He didn't know I was trying to protect him and us.

That experience has forever shaped me. I found the love a sexual pleasure, along with the feeling of being adored, and the fun of alcohol and food, and I spent my life trying to get that feeling back. I've heard that drug addicts are always looking for their first hit. I was always searching for that feeling again and it took me to a lot of bad places. I just wanted to feel safe, loved, and adored again. I craved that feeling that only Donny had given me.

As an adult looking back I know it was wrong. He was a man and I was a child. And I had already been groomed by a trusted older man. I was ripe for the picking.

But that is the point of why it was so profound for me. That experience was so inline with the contradictions of right and wrong, good and evil that I have spent a lifetime struggling with. It created the foundation of the Crap I needed to Unlearn.

* * * *

One day, someone I knew from high school invited me to hang out with him. I wasn't that close to him, I just kinda knew of him, so while it was strange that he was asking me to hang out, I could think of no reason why I couldn't, and I really didn't understand that I could say no, so I accepted.

We ended up at his friend's house, and that was when I met Dave. Dave was a cute older guy, and when he told my friend to leave us alone in his bedroom, and my "friend" did just that, I froze again when he forced me to have sex with him. I remember just laying there shocked, trapped, and unable to process what was happening.

I now know this to be date rape but that language didn't exist back then. This was long before the Me Too movement and I had been raised to believe in good girls and bad girls. I had already realized with those damn hoop earrings that I was one of the bad girls so I learned how to normalize traumas and abuses. I learned how to suck it up and suppress it. I learned how to find the safety for my mind in the midst of chaos. Little did I know then that this skill would lead to my eventual physical and mental disease. You can't carry poison in your body without being harmed by it.

But it happened, so I guess I was his girlfriend now, after all, we just had sex, and you don't have sex with someone who isn't your boyfriend, so now I had a boyfriend and tried to normalize this.

I will never forget the day that I brought my new "boyfriend" Dave home to meet my parents. My parents had taken me out to a local restaurant for dinner with a friend of theirs. They knew that after dinner they were going to meet Dave, and so they plotted and planned how this would go down.

Dave was the manager of an electronics store in the mall, and I think that was how they thought I met him.

As I am writing this, it occurred to me that maybe Dave had seen me in the mall and had arranged this meeting for me? I guess I will never know the answer to that but it is making sense to me now, in hindsight. Had I been brought to Dave as a sacrificial lamb? Had that "friend'" heard the rumors from high school that I was a slut?

My parents plotted and planned that they would grab a dining room chair and place it in the middle of the living room. They had a gooseneck lamp that they were going to place on the bookcase beside it so it could shine a light down on Dave, while they questioned him. During dinner, they planned their questions with so much fun, and the final question was going to be about whether he could get them a discount at his store.

My parents were having the time of their lives. When it was time to leave the restaurant, I needed to go to the bathroom, so my parents went to the car and moved it where I couldn't see it. I came out to join them, only to find their car gone. Here I was, the butt of their fun, while I was bringing my 'new boyfriend' home, and I was fed up and exasperated. I threw my hands up in the air and huffed. That's when I heard their laughter. The car was hiding around the corner, and they were watching to see my reaction to finding them gone. At least, they were having fun because I sure wasn't.

I called Dave and told them that he was going to be ambushed and he could back out of it. He said no, he could handle it. So, he came over, and he did handle it, and that made him acceptable to my parents.

Dave was there for my 19th birthday party. He was there when I was given a gold bracelet by my parents, and I can still see the picture of me in a pink and white striped mini dress, holding my hand out for him to clasp the bracelet on my wrist. I can see the picture of him at my surprise party that my friend Terry had planned for me with all my friends.

And then, I have no recollection of Dave again. He just disappeared.

I didn't miss the absence of Dave from my life. I don't actually remember much more about him. But the fact is that I had learned how to normalize rape rather than fight for myself, rather than hold myself to a higher standard. I betrayed myself by the very act of being silent. The way my brain was being wired by these events was creating patterns that were making it hard to distinguish between what was healthy or normal versus the reality I was experiencing. My desire to be accepted, to be loved, to be wanted would create a repeated pattern for me that when someone has sex with me, I let them into my heart and life, and then they are gone. That was how low my standards had become. Anything and anyone was better than noone.

That whole programming married sex with love and acceptance from an external source. Even to this day, even with all of the work I've done with my inner self, I still can't enjoy self-pleasure. It's just a release. I can't hug myself. I can't kiss myself. I don't know if self-pleasure will ever be "whole" or "natural," just because of all of my traumatic experiences around sex when I was younger.

* * * *

My father was so full of contradictions and contrast and so was his love for me. He would tell me over and over again that he loved me more than anyone else in the world, including my mother. I knew how much he adored and loved her so I equated his statements to the fact that I was unplanned and he was forced to grow up fast and become a man, a father, a husband and a provider. I know when I had my son, the very fact of my identity changing created something very unique in me.

But while he told me how much he loved me, I was also the one he took his anger and frustrations out on. He didn't handle a house full of females well; he didn't handle anything he thought was disrespectful well, and female teenagers who were as strong willed as me, appeared to be the straw that broke the proverbial back.

He would call me names, scream at me, and though he never struck me, he was physically abusive. That was a time when emotional intelligence was not known. He didn't know how to handle his emotions. Men were allowed only one emotion and that is anger. When my father was mad at me, he didn't know how to manage it and he would rage in ways that confused me.

One time he was so angry at my behaviour that he was shaking me by holding onto my hips and grasping my jeans. He shook me so violently that the fabric ripped. The fact that the fabric gave resulted in my falling down the stairs. Then we were at the store buying new school clothes and my sister asked why I was getting an extra pair of pants. My mother's response was, "Your father broke them." That was the only acknowledgement I received about that event.

Another time I was back talking to him while I was making myself a glass of chocolate milk. He was arguing with my mother about what I bitch I was being, and I wanted to fight back. He chased me, grabbed my drink, and lifted it to throw at me. I was trapped with a wall to my back and him at my front, and he let that glass fly. The glass didn't hit me, but it shattered everywhere, and I can still remember the spray of chocolate milk in a pattern around the walls.

How could he love me so deeply and still have so much anger towards me?

I struggled to understand what love was, how love and anger, or love and abuse, and how I could be treated so badly by everyone. It was beyond confusing. I realize now that it was that confusion that led to my inability to know the concept of boundaries and kept me in my bad relationships. If my father's deep love also included his anger and frustration, then I had come to see this as what love means.

I have learned that our brains are designed to make sense of things and we can normalize almost anything. It is built into our survival mechanisms that our brains will do anything in order to remain alive. I know this is how mental health issues like PTSD, schizophrenia and other issues are created. We can't live in perceived danger all the time, so we normalize our lives.

I know when my doctor was trying to find the source of pain and disease and would ask if I had abuse or trauma my answer was always an emphatic no. I had come to see all of this normal.

My Identity Changed

When I was 16 I was taken to a party with my friends. It was shocking to me that the party was hosted by one of our high school teachers. I guess he thought he was one of the cool ones and it was the end of the school year so he had the entire grade come to his home. He served us alcohol and there were kids everywhere. My best friend had taken up smoking and she offered me one.

I had always prided myself on not succumbing to peer pressure and so while I debated, I told myself I was old enough now and this was a choice and not being pressured. I took that first drag of my Players Light King Size cigarette and dragged that smoke deep into my lungs. I held it there and slowly exhaled as if I had been smoking my entire life. It was pure ecstasy to me even from that first drag.

I had no ability to stand up for myself to my parents so I hid things from them. While they and everyone else in my world were smokers, I was forbidden from smoking.

But I did.

So I hid it, like it was hideable.

I learned to lie because the truth was unacceptable. I learn to sneak around rather than having my parents be my support and structure. I hold truth and honesty to such a high value, I would rather lie than to see disappointment in her face. I would rather betray my own values in order to receive her acceptance.

When I was 21 I gave birth to my son as a single parent. I remember my mother being there for me during my labour. She was charged with getting my answers to the intake questionnaire for the hospital so when she got to the question about whether I smoked, I said, "Yes". She gave me her "look" and tsk tsk tsk.

When I came home from the hospital, I was staying with my parents. My mother had taken vacation time to help me adjust to being a mother. I adjusted extremely well and fast and was doing chores around the house. I was washing the bathroom tub on my hands and knees and my mother came and asked me if I was doing as well as she thought without smoking. She had informed me that I was not allowed to smoke around her so I might as well quit. It didn't matter that I was an adult.

When I got married at age 32 my wedding was ruined for me because of this. How can you sneak a smoke in a wedding dress? I ended up leaving the wedding early and changing out of my dress into a casual outfit that I had planned to wear the next day in order to get as many cigarettes into me as possible. My wedding pictures of my husband removing my garter belt are in a nice casual turtleneck set.

How can you feel aligned and proud of yourself when you are lying and sneaking around? How can you be fully empowered if the opinions of someone else dictate your choices and actions?

You can't.

Giving my power away to avoid my mothers disappointment was so destructive to my ability to live my life.

I would like to think that if my mother realized that it was her rules and her disapproval of my decision that pushed a wedge between us, she may have made different decisions.

That was another life lesson that would lead to my downfall. People pleasing and self denial in order to be labeled acceptable were a major part of my inability to take care of myself with honour.

* * * *

I fell hard for a man that I shouldn't have. He wasn't attractive but he was attentive. He made me feel like he thought I was the greatest thing ever to come into his world, so when his actions didn't match his words, I made excuses for him.

I became very good at creating stories for why people did the things that they did and those stories always made me feel better about the circumstances.

He was able to lead a double life, living with one woman and sneaking around behind her back with me and me not questioning his actions, just happy for when we had time for me.

I remember one day she called me and told me who she was. I was shocked and appalled. I had been seeing a married man for about a year and had no idea. She came over to my place and we talked for hours. She invited me back to her home where we could both wait for him to come home, while we compared stories.

When he opened the door and saw the two of us sitting there, you could see the shock on his face. He had been caught.

But he continued to get away with it because he had both of us under his control and neither one of us left him.

My personal standards had fallen to an all time low that I justified that I wasn't the one cheating and I would never be a cheater. To this day I have NEVER cheated on anyone but I did allow myself to be the other woman again. Because of all of the grooming that had happened to me, I had a belief system that I was only worthy of scraps. That didn't hide or remove the personal shame I felt in myself. The belief that I carried did not protect me from my shame.

At the age of 20 I found myself pregnant and alone. The father of the baby had disappeared and I chose to let him be gone. I had seen the damage that fighting could do to a child and if that is who he was, I let him.

Determined to rise up and be the best person that I could, I decided to keep my unplanned pregnancy. I vowed to my son that I would never let him pay for my mistakes.

After my son was born, I went back to school while on social assistance and worked on my business degree. Then I met the most amazing boy/man that I had ever known and I fell madly in love.

But even though I was using birth control, I found myself pregnant again. His parents begged me to terminate and let him get his career on stable footing. They told me how much they loved me and wanted me to be in their family but the timing was not right. They had accepted my son as their grandchild and I adored them.

I was sent to a doctor who obviously should never have been counseling women like me. I was 22 years old, a single mother of a one year old and my IUD had failed me. As he was examining me, he yanked the IUD out and showed it to me while spewing some nasty comments at me, as if I had lied about having one.

Against my better judgement, I allowed this doctor to perform the procedure on me. My boyfriend and his mother were with me during the pre-op and I was in so much emotional pain and turmoil. As they wheeled me away, I was sobbing so uncontrollably, that I was incoherent. I was trying to say stop, that I had changed my mind but it was too late, I was put under while I was crying.

When I woke up, I was not the same person. Something inside of me had died and I was never going to be the same.

I had made the decision based on my son and not wanting him to pay for my mistakes. I was willing to sacrifice for my son but forcing him to sacrifice for my actions was unacceptable to me. Keeping that pregnancy would have been forcing him to endure even less than my 100% because it would have been split between 2 that which wasn't enough for one.

I made the decision for the love of my boyfriend and his family and the acceptance and love that I felt from them.

I made the decision for my parents who had already become disappointed in me because I was an unwed mother and in their eyes had failed to reach my potential.

I made the decision for everyone but me. I went against myself, my beliefs, my core and I paid a high price.

I knew I was being punished when I found myself sick.

I was really sick and needed to be taken to the hospital. They found that there was still tissue inside of me and I prayed so hard that the procedure had failed and my baby was there.

He wasn't but infection had set in hard. I required another procedure to fix the mess that the previous doctor had left.

To this day, that man is the one that got away, the one I wonder what if...but our story was not going to end happily ever after.

I didn't handle the emotional pain of the abortion well. I didn't have the coping skills or the emotional strength to know how to deal with it all. I suffered from deep sadness and depression. I withdrew and our relationship was getting strained. In one of the deep moments of sadness I suggested we take a break from one another. He agreed and the break turned into forever.

I began to resent him deeply for my choosing him over my unborn child and then losing him anyway. It felt like the deepest betrayal even though I was the one who broke it off.

What if I hadn't terminated that child, would we have overcome the struggles and be happily married? What if we had counseling that helped us cope with the trauma and loss? We had just been sent home to deal with all those emotions by ourselves. Nobody ever asked us if we were ok.

Years later, when my son was a teenager and I was married with another child, I was exploring my spirituality, trying to fill the emptiness I felt. I went to a group meditation and we were guided into a deep trance. There I found my healing after that experience, all those years later.

My "child" was there meeting me in my trance. I knew it was him and I knew he was a boy. I felt him walk to my side and put his arm around my shoulder and hold me. I knew what he was saying but he wasn't speaking. It was unsaid but fully understood. He let me know that he had known that he wasn't meant for this world. That he fully supported and agreed with his short time in my life. He filled me with his love. I felt at such peace.

He had a purpose in my life and he had fulfilled it.

I could never have become the person that I grew into, without his sacrifice. I could not have loved and protected my children without knowing the depth of love and protection that I felt. He altered me forever.

I remember reading a book by Neale Donald Walsh called Conversations with God. It was a book I read during that time of my beginning of my connection with my own spirituality. In the book there was a little angel who offered to go to earth and be the opposite of what someone wanted in order for them to experience their goals. That was the first time I learned about the law of polarity and that everything must have a polar opposite in order to be experienced because without contrast, we have no relativity. In order to experience the light, it must be contrasted by darkness. In order to feel the depth of love, we must experience the loss of it or even hatred. Everything beautiful that we want in our lives can only be fully experienced through the experience of contrast and relativity.

I knew the son that I didn't bring into this world was my angel giving me my polar opposite to set me on the right path. I can't even comprehend who I would be, if anything else had happened.

Don't for a second think that this hasn't been one of the hardest things I have had to endure or that it was frivolous or easy. It was excruciating and yet I still believe in the power of choice and a woman's right to choose. What kind of person would I have been? Would I have damaged 2 other lives? The right decision for me has not been easy but it was part of my journey and I accept it.

And it was my decision to make.

My Heroes

I had 2 heroes in my life, one was my mother, and the other was my grandfather. I adored him. I was his first grandchild and he made me feel so loved. He had a prickly little mustache that went straight across his upper lip. He smoked Colts cigars and loved his beer.

My grandfather was very successful and self-made. He kept creating businesses and finding opportunities until and after he created his success. I remember as a teenager, I would go spend summers with them and do some really cool things. Every Thursday, we had to drive to downtown Toronto to go to the bank, where he would withdraw the weekly payroll in cash. My sister and I would sit in the car while my grandparents went in to do their business.

After we went to the bank, we had to go to a local hotel and go to their restaurant and have pie. My family life never included outings for pie in the middle of the afternoon, and it felt so decadent. I loved it.

After the pie, we would go back to his business which was called Baldwin Paper—man, did that make me love having the name Baldwin, seeing it up on that building. At the office, I would watch as my grandmother counted out the exact change to fill the payroll envelopes with cash for their employees. On the outside of those payroll envelopes were written in my grandmother's handwriting the deductions and how the amount was calculated.

One day, while sitting in a car in downtown Toronto, waiting for my grandparents to come out of the bank, I saw a helicopter in the sky. It had a heavy thing hanging from it, and it was swaying in the breeze. It was absolutely fascinating, and I was amazed. The helicopter was bringing the top sections of the CN Tower that was being built in my home city. The CN Tower is as iconic as the Eiffel Tower or the World

Trade Center in New York. I was literally watching history being made and the skyline of my hometown forever changing for the world.

My grandparents had the most fantastic home. It was a backsplit house, but it had 5 floors. The main level was the biggest entry I have ever seen in a "normal" family home. To the right was the formal living and dining room. I only ever went there once a year at Christmas. To the left was a huge kitchen. Up half a flight of stairs was the family room, laundry room, office, and guest bathroom. Up a full flight of open stairs were the bedrooms: 3 guest bedrooms, the main bath, and then the main bedroom with its own bathroom. From the main floor, you could go downstairs to the real family room where there was the bar, another massive guest bathroom, and down another half flight to the playroom.

This was where they had a jukebox that played 45 records. You would push a series of buttons, and the jukebox would rotate to that selection, and a mechanical arm would bring that record out and put it on the turntable and play it. I have so many amazing memories of my grandfather choosing "Ob-La-Di, Ob-La-Da" from the Beatles for us to dance to. He would grab my arm and swing me out so roughly that I would fly, and then he would pull me back just as hard. It was so much fun.

In that room, there was also a large pool table and pinball machines.

I can't tell how many memories remain with me in those spaces, but I can say they forever shaped my belief in family.

One moment that has never left me was a life lesson my grandfather tried to teach me. I wanted a car. I was about 16 or 17, and I wanted a car. I asked him to buy me a car. This is what he said.

"Kathy, I am going to tell you how you can get a car, so listen closely. I want you to go and get me beers from the fridge. I want you to sit on my lap and snuggle with me. I want you to give me kisses on the cheek and tell me how much you love me. Then, you tell me about the car you found, where it is, what it looks like, what color it is, what it smells like, how much it is, and you tell me you found the car you absolutely must have and if you don't get it, you will just DIE! Then, I will have no choice but to buy you that exact car."

I was shocked. That felt like manipulation. I said, "I can't do that, Grandpa." These are words that I wished I had truly understood the power of and immediately changed my mind.

He said, "Kathy, it is your choice. I just told you exactly how to get a car, what you do with that is up to you."

Damn that good girl. The girl with the rules of "shoulds"

My grandfather was trying to teach me the value of clarity in your dreams, how to see the details so clearly that it had to happen. He was teaching me about the universal law of manifestation and attraction. He was trying to tell me that when a man loves you like he loved me, that it would be impossible for him to say no to me. He was teaching me about the divine masculine being the foundation and strength. He was trying to teach me that I could have anything I wanted including true love and acceptance. He was trying to teach me that he wanted to be my hero and it was safe to let someone take care of me.

Why didn't I listen to how to visualize, how to find exactly what I want, how to make it crystal clear, and then how to stop at nothing until I get it? He tried to instill the true spirit of empowerment in me, but the crap that I had learned about what was right or what I was supposed to do was already deeply ingrained in me.

He tried to teach me how to be my authentic feminine self and have the security of the divine masculine but my choice led me to live a life where I was living logical, in control, in my masculine rather than the passionate, excited, creative feminine that I was born to be.

He knew it was in me, and he tried to get it out.

Grandpa, I am a late bloomer, but I heard you. I never forgot, and I never stopped trying.

* * * *

Every Christmas, the entire family would gather. My father was one of four children, and they all had children. It was a big, loud event when we got together every single Christmas Day. The dining room table was huge and had so many leaves in it that it could seat all the adults, and the kids' table was set up in the living room, yes, the room we never ever used except for then. Eventually, as I grew older, I was able to sit at the adult table.

We had to dress up for Christmas. It was special. So, I always wore an outfit that I had just received from opening my gifts on Christmas Eve. The table was always beautifully set with the china that had roses around the edges and crystal and silverware. There was also a small breakfast juice glass where we would be served tomato juice.

There was never a question of whether you were attending or not, you just knew that was where you were going to be, everyone would be there, and we were a large, loud, loving family. My grandparents were the glue, and they held us together tightly.

On one of those Christmases, I remember my grandfather talking about giving everyone in the family shares of the company. I was included in that, and I would be a director, and I would get a salary. When I asked what a director did, my grandfather said that once a year, I would have to come to a boring meeting and then go out for dinner with the family and get paid. It sounded like a great idea to me, and I was thrilled knowing that I was included in his vision for the company and the family.

That year, I remember my grandfather feeling so much love for his family sitting around the table that he said we have to do this more often, not just at Christmas.

While he spent time individually with his kids, it was only once a year that we were all together. He took my parents on trips with him, came to their home, and took them to local bars with live music. He was so gregarious that the band always came and sat at his table and became his friends.

He would invite the bands to come to his home and set up in the basement family room and play for a party. He made life exciting, possible, and contagious.

It wasn't long afterward that we went out for dinner as a family. We went to a restaurant, and it was like Christmas in the middle of the year. I asked my grandfather if I could order escargot. He told me absolutely not, they are gross. When I looked at my mother, she smiled and laughed, of course, I could have them, he was just being funny.

The next Christmas was our last. My grandpa got sick. He had lung cancer. I was never really filled in on the details. My dad was emotional but did not have the greatest emotional intelligence. He felt things so deeply and strongly but had no idea how to process or articulate those emotions, so he tended to be very reactive.

That year, we had a family gathering before Christmas. All I could see was my grandfather sitting on the sofa where he used to take naps cuddling with my grandmother, the sofa where I snuggled up and watched TV with him when I visited, and there my hero sat, obviously weak and sick. When we said goodbye, I reached down and kissed my grandfather, and my father flew into a rage.

He screamed at me. What was I doing? Was I trying to kill him? Didn't I know that any germ could be deadly to him?

I sobbed all the way home.

And that was my last moment with my hero. He died on December 26, 1984. I was only 19 years and my fairy tale family would not disintegrate with his passing.

* * * *

In Canada, December 26 is a holiday called Boxing Day. It is a holdover from British royalty where the servants were given the day off to spend Christmas with their families after serving the rich families for the actual holiday. In Canada Boxing Day used to be sacred. It was an extension of Christmas Day and everything was closed.

Some families celebrated with their extended family on that day, like Christmas Eve was for us. It was a day of peace and quiet. A day when only our immediate family was together. We played with our new toys, stayed in pj's all day, ate leftovers and just enjoyed the feeling of the holiday, without all the hustle and bustle. The world outside was paused and it felt safe like a cocoon.

I miss those days. Now it is still a statutory holiday but all the stores are open and it is pure consumerism.

Even though Boxing Day was the least significant in our house because the celebrations were over, it will always have a haunting significance for me.

* * * *

Our Christmas Eve took weeks to prepare. All of the silver came out one day, and the day was spent polishing it. Food was prepared for almost a week as we had what was called a cold table as our main meal. The meal was filled with small dishes of fatty fish, like smoked eel, smoked salmon, herring, etc. We had an Estonian dish of beets, herring, and potato salad that we called "the pink stuff". I loved that pink stuff. We had smoked turkey, smoked ham, and so many other delicacies. We would talk, laugh, and take small little helpings over and over again until we were stuffed.

(One year, my grandmother went to the Estonian house in Toronto and had a smoked turkey prepared. The turkey was smoked, the skin was peeled back, the meat was sliced beautifully, and the skin was replaced, making it look like it was an uncarved complete bird. It was spectacular.)

Then we would have the second course. That was blood pudding sausage, with pork belly slices, lingonberry sauce, and roasted potatoes. The sausage was dry and heavy, the pork belly was rich and fatty, and the lingonberry sauce was tart. Can you tell I love the combination of textures and contrasts of flavors?

We used to have a third course, but that had to be adapted. For many years, we then had a complete turkey dinner with all the fixings. That was in homage to my father and how he celebrated. My mother tried to make sure that everyone was always included.

I was raised with a lot of polite social rules, and one of them was to make sure that your guests were never left being the last ones eating. It would make them feel bad, so I learned how to eat past being full. I learned how to put others' feelings ahead of my own body and my needs. That would be another pattern of crap that I would need to unlearn one day.

Most of the guests at the table would serve food on our plates and move it around a little trying to be polite, and then ending up throwing all that food into the garbage because nobody had the capacity to put another morsel into their belly. Eventually, my father conceded, and we lost that last course. He didn't give up the turkey, though. My mother cooked the turkey the day before so we could have toasted turkey sandwiches in the middle of the night while opening presents.

All of this happened after we returned from the Christmas Eve candlelight church service. We weren't a religious family, even though my parents did the obligatory baptism of me and sent me to Sunday School at the local church regardless of the denomination. But Christmas Eve was different. It was a must.

When I was really young, we used to go to the Estonian church, but it was hard on my dad, my sister, and me. We didn't know the language or the songs. We just followed the crowd to keep my mother and her side of the family happy.

We didn't know the language because my father was Canadian for many generations. I still don't know if that side of the family goes back to Ireland or Germany or both, but either way, he was definitely NOT Estonian. My mother did not want him to feel any more isolated than he already did when my mom spoke her native language to her family in front of him, so we were not taught.

We were not sent to an Estonian camp because my mother witnessed as a child how the bi-racial non-pure Estonian children were treated, and she would not allow us to be subjected to that. (Prejudice is prejudice, no matter what it looks like, it still feels the same.) For me, that prejudice was ingrained deep in our family, and I knew that I was the bastard child who ruined my mother. I was never good enough because my father was never good enough. We were not purebred. My mother tried so hard to keep the peace and begged me to be nice because they were family. It didn't matter how they treated me or how I felt. Family came first.

Eventually, we went to a local English-speaking church where there was the singing of carols and the candlelight ceremony that felt like Christmas to my mother and comforting to my dad and me. Even though I am not a church fan, I loved those moments. I loved the songs and singing. I loved the feeling of community and connection. I loved dressing up in special clothes. I loved the feeling of family all together. I loved every single aspect and second. I miss how special those holidays were.

After church, we went home and enjoyed our feast. Near the end of our time celebrating Christmas like that, our traditions expanded. We began to have close family friends join us for dinner on Christmas Eve, so the event became even more special and connected. The opening of our gifts was at the end of the evening, BUT it couldn't begin until everything was cleaned and put away. You would have thought we were a hive of ants by how efficiently and quickly we put away those leftovers and cleaned the kitchen spick-and-span.

Santa was real in my home because Santa came to the house, and Santa gave us our presents sitting on his lap. There was no question about the magic because how could you deny the reality of hearing Santa's jingle bells and heavy footsteps above us? Or deny his jolly laugh as he ho, ho, hoed down the stairs to where we were waiting for his arrival. And how could you deny it as Santa gave each of the children their gifts and sat and enjoyed the process of opening each and every one of them?

Santa was very real and remains real to me. Not as a man but as a spirit. A spirit of giving selflessly, sharing joy, and creating magic.

When Santa and our guests left, we then got to the gluttony of opening our presents, and I mean gluttony. It was the 70–80s, and presents took literal hours to open. One year, we were opening gifts until 5 am, all the while eating sweets and cookies and toasted turkey sandwiches while the adults enjoyed copious amounts of alcohol.

Then, on Christmas Day, we would clean up the mountains of wrapping paper and bows, get dressed again, and head over to my father's side of the family. That was my happy Christmas. It was loud, it was messy, it was over the top, it was obligatory, and it was revered. Family was everything.

Boxing Day was the day that you played with your new toys, read your new books, and hung out all day in your new pajamas. It was quiet and restful.

Until that last Boxing Day of December 1984.

The day before, my grandfather had summoned up the last of his strength to open Christmas morning presents with my aunt and her family. When all the presents had been opened, he was ready and asked to be taken to the hospital.

Boxing Day, 1984, for me, is the memory of me, sitting on the stairs in the house I grew up in, waiting for my parents to walk in the door from the hospital and tell me that my grandfather had just died.

My world stopped, and I sobbed.

My father, who was devastated and overcome with his own grief, yelled at me to stop it, didn't I know how he felt? It was, after all, his father.

His funeral was New Year's Eve, and the viewing times were spread over 2 days prior to his actual funeral. Because he was so loved, and so connected, it took 3 days for everyone to come and pay their final respects. Those 3 days were the last days of us being a family, together. Our family never ever recovered from the loss of my grandfather.

I remember on one of the days between the afternoon and evening viewing at the funeral home we all went out to dinner together. We were discussing the details of the funeral. I was only 19, but I was old enough to be kind of respected as a contributing adult in the family. I remember suggesting that we play "Ob-La-Di, Ob-La-Da" at the funeral, and we all laughed and remembered and agreed, yes, that was a perfect song to play at his funeral.

New Year's Eve came and so did my goodbye to the man that I never envisioned ever having to live without. The funeral ended with the procession of cars driving down busy Toronto and me watching everyone stop and let us stay together in respect as we drove to the graveyard. There we said the final goodbyes, and I remember being so upset that we were leaving my grandfather in the coffin, in the cold, outside, and just walking away. I now know the ground was frozen, and he could not be buried until spring, but I didn't know how to deal with the emotions of just leaving him there.

While those 3 days of the safety of the funeral home, surrounded by all my family, were blessed for me, when it was over, I could not get far enough away. I had arranged to go to my best friend's mother's home for New Year's. Yes, the same mother that I told about my attempted rape; she was still who I ran to for full acceptance.

It was there that my healing from losing my rock began, and, at the same time, realizing that family was those that you chose, not necessarily always and only the ones you were born with. That was important for me to know because I had no idea how much family could hurt you at that point, but I was going to very soon.

My family was forever shattered and broken from that moment. My grandfather died without a will. I do not know if it was because he was arrogant enough to think he was immortal or that he thought he wasn't as sick as he really was, or if his jokes of letting them figure it out after he is gone were really how he felt. Whatever the reason, money changed everything.

The messiness of an estate without a will pit my family against each other. Siblings lost each other, cousins were divided, and that was the beginning of my full estrangement from my family.

When my grandmother died about 20 years later from Alzheimer's, I was asked to be a pallbearer. One of the other pallbearers was my cousin, whom I didn't know. I remember shaking his hand and introducing myself to this adult man that I was his first-generation cousin and I didn't know him.

That began the slow unwinding of my family. Death can break apart fragile bonds if not carefully honored and protected, and our family had already become accustomed to rejecting and abandoning each other rather than working through the difficulties that arose. For some reason it became normal and natural to just cut people out of your life, without a discussion, without fighting for the bond of family.

And I would endure loss after loss that would eat away and erode the person that I was and hone me into the person I am becoming.

I was raised in a world of 'what happens at home, stays at home.' And the secrets and pain that were unresolved would eat at the fabric of the family that I loved. I would systematically lose a piece at a time until I was alone and had a complete breakdown.

But I was strong and I pushed and pushed myself through every moment until I couldn't push anymore.

But the Universe was trying to talk to me, and I couldn't hear, or when I did, I would forget quickly. My body was trying to get my attention, but I ignored it and became physically sicker and sicker. My heart hardened. I attracted damaged, wounded souls to me and tried to save them, rather than focusing on myself. I became a walking magnet, attracting traumas, attacks, and simultaneous systematic rejection.

* * * *

I thought losing my grandfather was the only one that I would lose that was part of my core, but I was so wrong.

Betrayal and abuse come in so many forms and are incredibly damaging.

My sister and I are exactly 12 months apart. My mother conceived me at 15 because birth control was not an option for her at that time. She conceived my sister because she believed that she could not get pregnant while breastfeeding.

We were so close in age that it felt like we were raised as twins, except I felt so protective of her my entire life. I would follow her around, making sure she was safe, protected, and had everything she needed. As an adult, she was my best friend. We did everything together, and I could not love her more than I do.

My sister got married, had two children, and bought a beautiful house in the country. Her husband was self-employed and worked from home. From the outside, it appeared they had everything.

I, on the other hand, was a single mother, struggling to make ends meet, constantly broke, and in total contrast to her. Even though she had it all, I still gave her everything I had to give. When she asked me for something, the answer was always yes. So, when she asked me to babysit her newborn child, so she could attend the funeral of a friend, I, of course, was there for her. She had just given birth and was physically exhausted, and now the grief of losing a friend was a lot for her.

You know those moments in time when you wished you could go back and do things differently, this is my moment.

I would give anything to make different choices, different decisions, and create a different outcome, but I can't. So, I have to live with how I betrayed myself and betrayed her by keeping the traumatic abuse quiet that I suffered from her husband.

I told my sister to go to bed and sleep through the night. I would stay awake until her child had its midnight feeding, so she could get a full night's sleep. Everyone went to bed, and I settled into my nightgown and some TV, while the baby slept near me.

Shock doesn't come close to explaining how I felt when her husband came downstairs in his boxers, sat beside me, stroking himself and begging me to give him oral sex. He said he loved my sister and would never cheat on her, but he really wanted it.

Would I have not frozen if I had not had those previous experiences? Could I have had the wits to slap him in the face and run to tell my sister what atrocity her husband was trying to do right under her nose?

Woulda coulda shoulda.

I didn't. My brain froze. I was in total shock and panic. I stayed awake all night, terrified that I would be forced to physically fight him off. In the morning, I woke up my son and left quickly.

I could not face my sister. How could I hurt her like that? How could I tell her that her husband was the kind of person to betray her in her own home, right after she gave birth, thinking he was not cheating by begging her sister for sexual favors?

How could I handle admitting that I was seen as another object for men to do what they wanted with? Hadn't I already dealt with enough of that? Why wasn't I safe with my own family?

Here was another pattern that would take a lifetime to break and heal.

Men treated me any way they wanted.

And I allowed it.

I didn't believe I had a choice.

Maybe it started with Dave when I had him become my boyfriend after he raped me.

Maybe it started with the grooming by the neighbour and maybe I shouldn't have been swept away and lost my virginity to an older man when I was underage.

Maybe it started before I was born and I carried the shame of being unplanned.

Whenever or however it started doesn't really matter. This was the CRAP that I was living with.

I often wonder how differently me and my life would have turned out if the knowledge that I have now was common knowledge for my parents when I was born. I believe that I would not have been subjected to the kind of treatment that I experienced in every aspect of my life. I imagine living in healthy alignment with who I authentically am and what I could have accomplished rather than just surviving all those years.

I was existing in a world where I had no safety.

I had no sanctuary. And now, my brother-in-law had just built the first piece of the wall that would eventually tear my sister from my life.

It was a lot before the Me Too movement. Men thought that they could and did whatever they wanted, and I had no voice. My parents' friends would try to seduce me and buy me with money in order to have sex with them. At work, I would have to endure all sorts of crazy inappropriate abuse and had to just shut up and put up. I had an executive ask if I would run down the hall, so he could watch my breasts bounce. Or the manager who made me a cassette tape of seductive songs saying that he wanted me to know how he felt about me. Then there was an executive, who took me out for my birthday, told me I was safe with him, and then forced himself on me, while I lay there crying. I could recount the times male friends would force themselves on me or take me to a secluded park in a van. I could think about the men who pursued me until I relented and then dumped me. I can add to the pile of unsafe places in my home, my workplace, my school, on the streets, and now my own family.

That was a shock to my system that I was not going to process easily. That one was tough to stuff down and suppress.

The world was trying to tell me that I did not matter. That I was a thing to be used and tossed aside. So, it shouldn't have come as a shock to me that my brother-in-law told me to grow up and let it go, because his wife kept bugging him about why her sister was so distant.

My parents pushed me to tell them the truth because they could see so clearly that something had happened and then told me that because I didn't say anything then, I had to just keep it quiet, keep it to myself, and deal with it. They were trying to protect me, my sister, and the family, and the 'don't talk about it' rule was rooted deep in our family.

I had become an expert at suppression and putting on a happy face. I had become an expert at hiding the truth and putting my big girl panties on. And my expertise was killing me.

I was unable to resume an in-person relationship with my sister until I was with my soon-to-be husband. With him at my side, I could visit my sister and not have to worry about another sexual assault. But I also put that burden of carrying the secret on my man. I forced him to never let anyone know what had happened. I did not understand the ramifications of his keeping my promise. I did not realize that I was robbing both of us of his standing up and being my man, my protector, and how damaging it was to him to pretend this horrible game of a normal happy family.

I did not realize or know that my husband had his own family burdens and secrets that he carried, and my forcing him to carry mine was destroying his soul.

I lost my newly married husband the day he lost his mother. She had been denying her body, so it was failing, and she was getting sicker and sicker since before I came into their life. She refused to go to a doctor until it was too late. By then, we had married and were living a life where we were both finding ourselves. We had both suffered job losses due to other people's decisions, we had lost our savings in the stock market, and we were coming together as a new family: my husband, my son, and I.

My mother-in-law died on December 23, 1995, 11 years after my grandfather and at Christmas again. She died with regrets, knowing that she had let fear keep her from her dreams, facing her illness, and truly living, and now it was too late. One of the last things she said to me was, "I don't want to die, and now it's too late."

We made her final arrangements on Christmas Eve. Her final wishes were to make sure that her body was cremated and make it as cheap as possible. I will never forget the guilt that the funeral home put on us when we shared her request and they had us look at the cardboard box that she would be cremated in. As if it mattered to her or to us. Only the funeral home would see her in it. Why did they feel they needed to guilt us into purchasing a more expensive box for their profits? When do business and humanity become one?

We left the funeral home and went to celebrate Christmas with my parents. We forced ourselves to put our grief behind us for a day and participate, but Christmas was really beginning to lose its magic and glory for me. It would take more circumstances to add up, but eventually, I would get to the place where I wish that Christmas did not exist. I would eventually dread the holiday and wish that I did not have to participate in a tradition that just caused me pain for the sake of others' happiness, for tradition, and for a religion that was not mine.

When she died, a part of my husband died, too. I lost the man that I married emotionally, but we would push through for another 16 years of torturing each other with our damage, our past, and our pains until we could no longer do it.

My relationship with my sister was strained, but we persevered, and somehow, I could be in the same room as my brother-in-law without screaming, but every time I looked at him, we both had this horrendous secret between us, and I hated being bonded to this man through secrecy and betrayal.

Secrets kill. They destroy. I have had to deal with a world without a horizon for most of my life. Hiding the truth from everyone, carrying their burdens, their secrets, and being their cover for the world.

I had to be the bitch, so others could be the heroes and hide their pain. I had to hold the world steady for everyone around me while mine was falling apart. I had to watch people I love lie to my face and make me think I was the crazy one, while their secrets, their pain, and their addictions ate away at my soul.

* * * *

My parents retired to Mexico and took my mother's mother with them. They retired early as they had capitalized on stock trades and the increased value of their assets. They had a plan that would allow them to live off the interest of the portfolio without ever having to touch the principal and live happily ever after.

That was their plan, but it was not their reality. Their actual reality took their lives in their prime, after long battles of addiction and disease. Their reality cut them off from their family, friends, and support system because they lived in the time before FaceTime, Skype, or Zoom, which make long-distance connections possible and sustainable in today's world. Their plan did not include the emotions, the beliefs, the need for security and comfort, or how we are hardwired as people.

Their plan was flawed, and I carried the burden when it failed.

But those years also gave me profound life lessons that have forever changed and affected who I am. Since I learned my lesson that my grandfather tried to give me when I was a teenager, I learned to identify when a life lesson arrived and take it.

When my father's mother died, and we were reunited as a family, it should have been a sign. My parents were living in Mexico, and they flew up for the funeral. The flight was paid for by the family business that my grandfather built. The estate was still a contentious, unresolved issue, still plaguing the family, but at least they were here.

This was the first time I had hosted my parents in my own home. They stayed with me because their relationship with my sister was broken since they moved away. This funeral would bring all broken relationships to a head, and there would be fallout.

I had my own issues as my husband had worked for my brother-in-law, and his pay was not what was discussed when the original agreement was made. We felt trapped by family obligations, and my husband and I worked harder and harder to make ends meet. We would borrow money in the form of a pay advance, and then my husband would work day and night, 7 days a week, to pay it off. It was a vicious cycle, like being trapped in payday loans, but it was complicated by family. I cleaned their home for years rather than paying a cleaning lady to pay off those payday loans. I carried the shame of scrubbing my sister's toilets like I was Cinderella, all because we could not make enough money and keep family relationships at the same time. We would do anything to get ahead of this and finally break the dependency cycle we felt trapped in.

The relationship between my sister and I finally broke when my brother-in-law called to put me in my place. As he tried to control me and manipulate me, I yelled at him, how dare he talk to me like this when I have kept his secret all those years. It was obvious at that moment that my sister was able to hear every word. I could feel her punched in the heart. My brother-in-law said he would tell her everything as soon as we got off the phone.

The next day, my sister told me her heart had been broken, and we shall never speak of this again.

And that was the end of my having a sister. It's a loss that I still hurt from today, but one that I have learned to live with.

And that was the end. I no longer had a sister. It's a huge source of pain for me today, but I have learned to cope with my loss.

* * * *

So, here I was, hosting my parents in my home, while I worked at a local grocery store for a minimum wage because we lost our income and our credit, and couldn't afford to pay our car insurance. I had been building a direct selling business, and without a car or insurance, I just snuck away and hid in my embarrassment and shame.

My husband was rebuilding himself with a new job and career, and it required that he travel an hour to work, driving the backroads so as not to be pulled over by the police. We were hanging on by a thread, and our relationship was suffering.

So, there we were, my parents and I, in my backyard, sitting on their old outdoor furniture where so many memories were woven into the fabric, when the gasman walked into my backyard and turned off our gas. Our bill was past due, again. We were trapped in a cycle of robbing Peter to pay Paul, and we were not winning.

It was beyond humiliating for me to face my weaknesses at such a vulnerable time as a funeral, especially when this was the first time in years I had been with my parents. We were all coming face-to-face with the shards of broken glass that once was family, and I was doing it while showing how broken and a failure I had turned out to be.

My entire life felt like I was trying to prove myself, to be worthy and to capture the respect and attention of my parents, especially my mother. Here I was showing my darkest failure and the irony of the moment was so profound.

My mothers shock and disappointment was so apparent it was written all over her face.

My father took me to the local wire transfer location in our local grocery store. There I had him pay for my outstanding amount so we could all resume having hot showers. It was $600 and it might as well have been a million for me.

Part of me was so relieved that my parents were there to support me. I never felt that I was that important to them. My parents had always supported my sister. She got the wedding paid for. She got the showers. She got the diamond earrings for her wedding present. She got the housewarming gifts.

I never did.

This moment of my falling and my father supporting me actually made me feel safe and appreciated. Unfortunately that feeling didn't last. Months later as I was just getting myself back on my feet, my dad was pressuring me to pay him back.

Another fall.

* * * *

We all carry our demons, and one day, my mother had way too much to drink, and she poured her heart out to me. We sat, two women, both with our pains and traumas, and tried to be there for each other. She said something that day I will never forget.

"Kathy, you don't understand. I could have been somebody."

On the surface to the rest of the world, she looked like she had it all. She was young, successful, and beautiful. They had retired to Mexico in their 50s. But inside, I know she had lost dreams, lost passions, and lived her life based on the circumstances and expectations of others and society. She did not live aligned with her greatness. She felt that she had failed, and depression, anxiety, and alcohol took her soul.

That day I knew somehow I had to figure this out. Somehow, I had to make sure that I never died with my dreams still inside of me, with gifts unfulfilled, and feeling like I had given up. I had seen too many people die with regrets, damage, and baggage left for others to carry and clean up. I knew I had to do better, but I was still trapped in my own crap, and that day was not then. I would still have more to fall before I could find the strength to reverse that free fall I was experiencing myself.

* * * *

I visited my parents about a year after that. I went and stayed with them for about 3 weeks, and I am so blessed to have had that time. My mother had fallen and broken her hip, and she was recovering from the surgery when I was there. They wanted to show me the area and show me this new home that they had come to love, but my mother felt restricted by her pain. That meant that my father and I had a lot of time alone to explore.

My father and I had a difficult relationship my entire life. We were too much alike. We could easily push each other's buttons and bring the worst out in each other. He loved his CB handle, 'The Captain', and it fit his personality. He wore captain hats, wore t-shirts with Captain on them, and had this sign that said...

**To the crew, Please be reasonable and
do things my way. Signed the Captain**

We were trying to forge a new relationship as adults and it was beginning with this visit.

There was one destination that my parents really wanted me to see, but I insisted that my mother come along. She really did not want to because of the pain in her hip, but she finally agreed. The trip was a couple of hours, and her sitting in one position in the car was beginning to take its toll on her. When we arrived at this beautiful place, high on a mountain in Mexico, in a small quaint town, my mother lifted her leg to get out of the car, and it got stuck in position. She was frozen in pain, in a literal purgatory of halfway in the car and halfway out of the car. And the pain was excruciating.

I tried to help. I tried to make suggestions but everything I did just seemed to make the situation worse. Out of frustration, I could not control my own tears, and my mother snapped at me to stop it.

I did. I sucked it down, and my mask came back on. All I could think to do was go on a search for a doctor who could help. In my broken, non-existent Spanish, I managed to find a doctor who could communicate enough to write a prescription for a couple of strong painkillers. I found the pharmacy, got the pills, ran back to the car where my mother was suffering, and gave her the pills. She took them, and within minutes, I could see the relief of them taking effect and her face relaxing. She was able to get her leg back into the car, and we reversed our trip and went back home. The only part of that quaint town I saw was the shops and clinic, looking to help my mother.

When we got back to their home, my mother told me that when there is a crisis, I can't be part of the solution if I am in the depth of the problem. I was of no use to her if I was crying and feeling my own pain.

I remembered when my mother-in-law was dying, and the hospital had called and said come now, that I had reached out to my mom. During that difficult time, while I was waiting for my husband to pick me up and bring me to the hospital, my mother asked if I wanted her to just talk fluff or to let me cry. I asked her for the fluff, and it grounded me.

I knew what she meant about how you can help someone only when you are not in the depths of the pain with them. There needed to be distance from the emotions, or your brain could not function properly. That was one of my first lessons in truly understanding the power of our central nervous system.

That visit was the last time I saw my mother in person, but it was not her last lesson for me. Her last lesson came after her death.

One day, I was woken up by the phone ringing. When I answered and heard my father's voice, I immediately knew something was wrong. My dad did not call me, he did not call me early in the morning, and he sure did not call me to chat. Skype had just come to be, and that was how we spoke, so I knew something bad had happened.

My father asked me if I was sitting down. In my fear and exasperation, I said you just woke me up, I am in bed, yes I am sitting down.

That's when he told me that my mother had died in the middle of the night.

WHAT? WHAT?

It took me a few seconds to wrap my brain around this concept.

My mother was dead. She was gone, and she was only 58.

As I write these words, I can't help but notice that I am 59. I am now a year older than my mother ever got to experience.

Shock does not come close to what I felt. She had just had surgery for a stomach ulcer. The surgery had been a success. She had just come home the night before. How could she be dead?

I have no idea how I did it, but somehow, I booked a flight immediately to Mexico, leaving that day. I told my dad I was coming, and even though he protested, I know he was relieved. His one and only, the love of his life, was gone, and he was really sick himself. I knew that, but I didn't know how bad it was.

Once the flight was booked, I tried to reach my sister. I called and called but got no answer. I ran out of time trying to find her before I needed to get to the airport and fly away.

I rushed into the airport, checked in, got to my gate, and now I was left alone with nothing but my thoughts and grief. With as much grace as I could muster, I made my way to the ladies' room and fell on the floor sobbing like a fox caught in a trap. If you have never heard that sound, it can be compared to a woman being raped, fighting for her life in sheer terror.

I guess it's not usual to find broken hearts and grieving people in emotional turmoil at the airport because everyone just walked past me as if this was normal. There was nothing normal about losing my mother when I was only 43 years old. She was 16 when I was born. I had always dreamed of being two little old ladies together.

This was not "supposed" to happen.

I was alone— just me.

No sister for help and support.

No mother, ever again. She was gone.

I was alone.

Suck it up, Buttercup! Put on your big girl panties. You have to be strong.

My husband called and told me that he found my sister while she was on vacation and had informed her of our mother's passing. My mother died thinking that my sister hated her. I know this because the last words I ever spoke to my mother were her asking, "Why, why does your sister hate me so much?"

I had no answers, and that is not the last words anyone should have to remember about a loved one.

While I was flying, my mother's body was being cremated. In Mexico, a cremation happens immediately after death unless the body is to be preserved for a casket funeral. My mother's wishes were to be cremated, so that happened without my being able to say goodbye.

When I landed, my father's neighbors had picked me up. It was the first time in my life that I landed in an airport to be met with a sign with my name on it. They took me to my father, and he was awake even though it was 11:30 at night. Just that morning, my father had called me to tell me that my mother had died, and there I was in the evening.

I can only imagine how my father was holding up. His wife died in the middle of the night. He had to tell her mother and daughter that she was gone, and he had lost his rock and his foundation. He had to then get to the funeral home and say goodbye to her, take care of his mother-in-law, and wait for me.

That alone was enough to make him look as haggard as he did, but I could see the physical effects of his own illness on him as well. It was shocking and scary as hell.

That night we stayed up late, and he told me everything. Every single detail. This was truly the first time in my life that my father was talking to me like an adult, an adult that he respected and trusted, and I was to learn the darkness of my mother's passing.

When we rose the next morning, and reality was beginning to set in, I was trying to get the lay of the land. My mother had lists of what he ate, what his vitals were, and what his schedule was. My father was having dialysis because he was in end-stage renal failure from his type 2 diabetes. I had to be his set of hands and help him with his healthcare regimens. He had a shunt surgically implanted that allowed him to give himself his own dialysis at home. The shunt attached to a bag that drained the poison from him. He needed to do this every couple of hours.

I was trying to figure out how to help him, get him fed, and be there for my 94-year-old grandmother, all the while still stuck in my role as a dutiful daughter doing as she is told while trying to suppress my own grief.

Right or wrong, suppressing my grief was my solution. It was the only tool I had in my emotional toolbox.

I muddled through the best I could and when I went to bed spent and exhausted that first day, I looked at a picture of my parents that had been taken while they were on a cruise. My mother was beautiful, strong, and smiling. They cuddled together, in love, and living life.

I looked my mother in the eyes of that picture and spoke to her. "Mom," I said, "I'm lost, I do not know what to do. How do I step into your place, how do I help Dad, am I the daughter, or am I now the adult caregiver? Help me." I pleaded and then fell asleep.

I woke up in the middle of the night or really early in the morning, and at first I thought maybe it was a dream. It seemed real but also not real, but I knew something life-changing was about to happen. I could feel my mother's breath on my ear, and I was filled with anticipation.

Then she spoke, and her message was crystal clear...

and I heard her clearly tell me...

Kathy, you know damn well what to do. Just do it.

I used to call my mother The Queen Bee because she was always telling me what to do. I used to resent when she did this. I used to feel like it was disrespectful. And this was the last thing she would ever tell me to do. It was as if she was passing the torch, telling me to trust myself, that she believed in me, but in her bossy strong voice so I knew it was really her.I can't tell you how much I had her to boss me around every single day. I can't express how much I miss her pissing me off.

When my dad woke up, I told him what had happened and what my mother had said. He looked at me and said, "Do what you think is right.

If you step on my toes, I will say 'ouch,' and we will deal with it together."

Where was this man and this attitude my entire life? 'The Captain' has surrendered his reign and his control, and now we could heal.

I spent 2 weeks with him, even though I had only booked a flight for one week. It was so obvious that I couldn't leave him that soon. He wasn't ready. So, I stayed, and my husband, who was now a long-distance truck driver, took our daughter on a week-long road trip that I don't think either of them will ever forget.

That extra week with my father made all the difference to him, his health, our relationship, and so much more. I asked my dad stories about his life, pulling as much of his life, his memories, as much as I could while we were together.

My dad asked me how he would live without her. And he meant it. She had been by his side since he was a teenager. They had loved each other and only each other for their entire lives. I told my dad he would need to create a new normal, and he tried. He really did try, even with his failing health and a broken heart.

One day, the funeral home arrived with a box filled with my mother's ashes. Another moment of stark reality had just hit home. My dad confessed that although he and my mom had discussed what they wanted to happen with their bodies when they passed, they never discussed what to do with the remains.

I took this time to have a serious end-of-life conversation with my dad. What did he want when his time came? He told me that he definitely wanted to be cremated, and he wanted me to use the funeral home as my mother, and then scatter his ashes in the Caribbean. That was not what I would ever have guessed. He couldn't swim, but he was 'The Captain.'

I promised him that when the time came, if he had not made any decisions with my mom, I would scatter their ashes together in the Caribbean. We discussed his will, and he made me the sole beneficiary. He wanted me to have everything, but it came with a condition. The condition was to promise that I would never make my grandmother move. That she could live out the rest of her life in the new home she had created right there in Mexico.

Little did I know, the weight of making end-of-life promises was heavy—very heavy.

I tend to give advice to those who are preparing for their own passing and help them understand the weight of their wishes on those they leave behind. Passing on their burdens is a heavy load to carry.

It took me years to fulfill my father's wish to scatter their ashes in the Caribbean. I was too busy fulfilling his deathbed promise of caring for my grandmother and my family.

But I finally did when I went on a cruise.

After my divorce, I began dating again. He invited me to join him on a Mediterranean cruise and my first response was "can I bring my parents?" He was confused. What on earth did I mean?

I shared with him my promise to my dad, and showed him the box with their ashes. Of course they could come. He even became my hero and offered to open their wooden urns, divide up their ashes and bring a portion of both them. He made jokes about them meshing together, that took such a traumatic event for me and remember the light and laughter that they shared. My parents aways had a strong physical, sexual tension in their entire marriage and now that was how they were being laid to rest.

We prepared to go the cruise and my partner offered to take care of the ashes. I felt so protected and cared for. We arrived at the airport and went through security, when I was shocked that we were being pulled aside. I always sail through security and now I was being questioned about the contents of my carry on bag. I realized that my parents were inside our bag. I was unaware. My parents' ashes were being taken care of for me so it was not in my consciousness.

I immediately panicked. I knew that security threw out anything that was not able to go past the checkpoint. I had images of bottles of water being thrown in the trash and all I could think of was that my parents were going to be discarded into the airport trash. I was terrified and horrified and immediately panicked.

My partner stepped up and explained the situation to security. He had packed their ashes in a bag and placed that safely in a shoe so that there was no chance of the bag breaking open and we could safely deliver them to their final destination.

What we didn't know was that we are supposed to inform security ahead of time when you are carrying ashes. What we didn't know was that human remains, without the 80% liquid that makes up the human body, the ashes become dense and appear to be solid to an x-ray machine.

Thank goodness we made it through security and arrived at the cruise. I kept looking at every angle location through the lens of is this the right place? Is this the right time? Is this what they would want? This was a serious once in a lifetime, unalterable decision that I had to make.

I kept looking for the right place and finally found it in Saint Martin. I had made the decision on the ship that I was going to purchase a ring of Tanzanite at the place where their ashes were scattered. I would know it was the right place, when I found the right ring.

I found a beautiful ring there that is shaped like a triangle. I liked the symbol of the 3 sides, mom, dad and me. Both sides of the stone are surrounded by a line of diamonds that feel like being surrounded by them and their love forever. I wear that ring on the finger beside where I wear my mother's wedding ring. My parents are never far from me, from my mind and my heart. I miss them more than I could ever adequately explain. It is guttural.

* * * *

Before I left my father in Mexico to return home to my husband and daughter, my father had one final request for me. "Would I please wash my mother's dying blood out of their mattress?"

I got a bucket and soapy water with a brush. I removed the bed sheets, and there were the remains of my mother, her last struggle, a pool of blood soaked into the mattress.

This was to be my goodbye to her. She had bled to death in her bed from internal hemorrhaging. She hemorrhaged because she could not resist drinking and getting drunk after returning home from ulcer surgery.

Her addiction was too strong. She couldn't fight it, and I wonder if she even wanted to.

She was struggling for so long with her depression and her lonliness, and now my dad was at the end of his life. Did she have what it took to go on without him? Was she paving the way for him to come to her? Their doctor had told me that he had seen countless cases of couples where the healthy one died just before the sick partner.

And now, it was again my mess to clean up.

I scrubbed and scrubbed. I kept thinking about that line from Shakespeare's *Hamlet* about her trying to get the blood out. I sobbed, I cried, I grieved.

It was hard work. She had left a lot of her behind. When I was done, my dad came and thanked me, and then commented on how wet I had made the bed. We had done enough healing by this time that I looked at him and firmly said, "Don't!"

He understood immediately.

When I went home to my house, that was when my world came crashing down on me. I was really being tested. I found out the lies that my husband had been keeping from me all these years. I found out all his secrets, and I was shattered.

I wish I could share with you the true depths of despair and true utter anguish I was experiencing, but there is no value to you, the purpose of this book, or me and especially to my family. So I am purposefully choosing to keep the details private.

Seriously, how much could a person truly endure?

I had known for a long time that our marriage was in trouble. We had been drifting for years since his mother died, and we were buried under the weight of debt, family, work, and exhaustion. But I had married him, and I had promised him until death do us part and I was determined to keep that sacred vow.

Now even my marriage and my husband was being taken from me.

My husband and I were fighting over the phone with everything unwinding in front of us. In the midst of this chaos, my father called. I told him, "I'm sorry, I can't talk right now."

Even though he had his own issues and pain, my dad knew when I was in crisis myself. He wasn't going to take no for an answer, and I think he found his old self, the father, not the sick, broken man again for a moment because that is what it sounded like to me.

And I needed a parent. I needed a support system. I had endured more than I could handle, and this explosion had taken me down. I told him everything. I told him the secrets, the lies, the effects on me and on my marriage, and how it was all over.

And my dad calmly said, "Your husband is a good man. Stay by his side and heal it"

While it took years after that for my husband and I to finally end our marriage, I did stay, and we did work on it together. We faced our demons, put all the cards on the table, and worked hard to clean up the mess we found ourselves in. That would never have happened if my dad did not give me those words of wisdom.

My husband is a good man, and I know that I am a good woman. Our marriage was needed for each of us to face our crap and bring it through a healing process. I realize that not all marriages or relationships are meant for life until death do us part. Sometimes we get into these marriages or relationships, and they are just meant for a season, a reason, and we put judgements and conditions like the contract of marriage.

My dad and I spoke several times a day. We became friends. I was there for everything he needed, and he was there for me. We had a profound healing those last 7 weeks of his life, and unfortunately, that was all the time we had. I had 2 weeks with him after my mom died and then 4 weeks over the phone.

My father had recently been admitted to the local clinic because he had an infection. Somehow his stint had become infected, and it was becoming dangerous. During that time, my dad had made sure everyone knew I was his next of kin, his decision-maker, and he had been giving me his instructions daily on what he wanted, and how he wanted it, and I was there for him. Even in the hospital and clinic, we talked every single day.

Our last week was in person but not in a good way. I got a call from his doctor, telling me I needed to come now. He needed a decision-maker.

I told the doctor that I had already booked a flight for next week because I needed to get my passport updated as it was about to expire. He told me that I had no time, so I booked a one-way ticket and headed back down immediately.

The doctor told me when I landed not to go to the house, but to get a taxi and go immediately to the hospital. Freaking out, I did exactly as I was told. I landed, grabbed a cab, and went flying into the hospital, looking for the ICU department.

The ICU was locked. There were specific visiting hours, and I was told I would have to wait. So, I sat for hours in the hallway, with my suitcase, waiting to be let in. Nothing made sense if I was told to rush there immediately but then told to wait until the appropriate visiting time.

When I was finally able to see my father, he looked at me and said, "Thank God, you are here. They took my wallet. Get my wallet, get my bank card, and here is my PIN." That one moment saved me more problems that were to arise in the future. All that information had been highly secreted, but my parents, who were responsible for my grandmother, who at 94, had no idea how to access her own funds. Her financial future was tied directly to that moment of sharing confidential information of a PIN number.

My father was stable. I had seen him. It wasn't required for me to be there every single moment, and I was sent home. I took another cab on the long road to my parents' home. I had to tell the cab driver how to get there because it was outside of the city. Thank God, I had just been there and knew the lay of the land. I arrived at the house, and the security guard at the gate knew who I was and let me in. I got into the house and walked over to where my grandmother lived. I startled her when I showed up at her glass door in the dark of the evening, but when she saw it was me, she was immediately relieved. She had been alone while my father was admitted, and she was confused and totally powerless. She needed to be cared for in every way except her personal care. Even at 94, she still cooked, cleaned, gardened, read, and loved her hockey.

She knew she was safe. She knew I would take care of her and my dad. She knew he was dying. You don't get to be 94 without being strong.

My father had driven his burgundy Lincoln Town car to Mexico. He had driven it down from Canada and while Mexico has a lot of paved roads, there are still a lot that are cobblestone roads. That boat either floated or bounced around. I was never allowed to drive it. Even when I came down after my mom died and I was the caretaker, my dad had his arm in a sling, he still refused to let me drive.

But now I had to get back to the hospital. I had no choice but to drive his car for the hour-long drive back to Guadalajara. When I arrived the next morning, he never asked how I got there. He was never told that I was now driving his beloved beast that nobody but he drove.

When I went into the ICU the next day, I had a couple of my dad's friends with me. He wanted to ensure that his will was signed and witnessed. He wanted to make sure his dying wishes were taken care of. I was the first to go into his room, and I was shocked, death was written all over him. I knew what it looked like, I had been with my mother-in-law while she passed, but it still shook me to my core.

When I came out of the ICU and sent the next friend in, I broke down in hysterics. I sobbed uncontrollably. A woman, a stranger, came to me and held me. She just grabbed me and held me. She kept talking, and I heard the Spanish word for Jesus, so I knew she was praying for me. She held me and prayed until it washed out of me, and I was okay again. And then, she just left me as quickly as she had arrived.

One of my dad's friends that I had brought was a retired nurse. She witnessed the whole thing. She said, "I thought you were prepared for this." I replied, "I thought I was, too."

He was scheduled for surgery. His shunt needed to be removed. It had broken inside of him and was making him septic. Not a good situation for someone already in renal failure.

I made the doctor's promise, no heroics. He was dying already. There was no need to extend his life just because... he was not getting out of this. We all knew it, we had all discussed it. My dad knew it, and he was ready.

I called my sister and told her the gravity of the situation. Even though we hadn't spoken in years, and she had cut my parents and me out of her and her family's life, I still was not going to deny her or my father's last moments. She made arrangements, and she would be coming down.

I was with my father as he was leaving for surgery. I told him that I was on my way to get my sister, and even though there was so much pain between their estrangement, he said, "That's good."

That's good. Those were his last words to me. He knew my sister and I were there for him, and he went into surgery.

Unfortunately, my dad crashed during surgery, and the doctors said they had no choice but to put him on life support. I was furious. How could they do this? Why didn't they let him go? We had discussed this prior, but the doctors said they were ethically bound because it happened during surgery.

My dad was unconscious and never regained consciousness again. He became stabilized by the life support machines, and now I was in the position to make the decision to take him off. I asked the doctors what the process would entail, and they said that once he was off life support, it would be less than 4–6 hours, and he would pass peacefully.

They didn't know my dad. They didn't know the strength of a Baldwin. That was not what happened.

My dad was moved to a single room, and while he was being moved, I went and paid the hospital bill. I made sure that I was clear that I wanted to pay for everything now. I did not want to make payments after his death as it would feel like I paid for his death.

His vitals began to fall, and it looked like the time was near. My husband arrived and asked for private one-on-one time with my dad. I don't know what he said to him except that I know he thanked my father for believing in him and supporting him during our crisis.

And then the death watch wait began. His blood pressure fell to 60/40, and he stabilized again. I stayed by my father's side. I slept on a cot in his room. I held his hand. I talked to him.

Every time a nurse came into the room, I would ask for the "numero" because that was all we could do to communicate, and somehow, knowing his stats made me feel some sense of control.

At one moment, I looked at my dad, and a tear fell softly from his eye. I knew he was aware and trapped inside his own body.

After 24 hours, the doctors told me to go home and not come back until he passed. They believed he was holding on while I was there. Against everything I believed in, I left, and I carried my father's cell phone, waiting for the doctor's call to tell me he was gone.

When the call finally came, my husband and I drove back to the hospital. Even though he died in the hospital, the mortician made me identify his body as he was being taken for immediate cremation. That is cruel and unusual punishment, in my opinion, but I have big girl panties, and I yanked them up high.

After his body was released to the mortician, I thought I was free to go, but it appeared that I had an outstanding bill to pay. My father had stayed past his balance owing and now the piper wanted to be paid.

Now, it was my time to keep my deathbed promises and try to create my own new normal.

* * * *

When both of my parents passed away, my marriage was in a massive crisis, and I was now responsible for my 94-year-old grandmother. It made perfect sense to me to sell everything that I own, move to Mexico, and care for my grandmother as I promised.

I mean, that is the logical, sensible thing to do when your world is crashing around you: make major life-altering decisions, isn't it?

This is one of those decisions that, if I knew how my central nervous system worked, how grief and stress cut off your ability to access your pre-frontal lobe, and that logical decisions are not possible because your brain has been hijacked by stress, maybe things would have turned out differently. But I didn't know, and it would be a long time before I figured it out.

The problem with my being strong, passionate, and responsible, along with unresolved trauma and disempowering beliefs and habits, was that I could push myself past any point of reason. That said, 'when the going gets tough, the tough get going' was truly me. I never stopped to process. I never looked for other solutions. I just took on the responsibility and life that my parents left in their passing.

I had been in the process of building a business with an idea that I was passionate about before I lost my parents. I believed in the connections of people, and I was feeling a great social divide happening because of social media. People were speaking online and the personal connections were becoming superficial. I thought if we could connect with people based on our own personal interests by meeting online and taking it in person, we could really make a difference in our personal lives. I called it "Feast of Friends." I loved the idea that would create our own personal feast of friendships that fit different aspects of ourselves.

Great idea, isn't it?

I was funding the building of this business with my own savings and kiting money from our household budget. The internet was new. Social media was new. Google was new. Everything about this was new. I hired coaches and programmers and learned everything that I needed to make it happen. And I worked and worked and worked.

So when I decided to move to Mexico in order to care for my grandmother, my thought was that I could continue to build this business, care for her, put my daughter in bi-lingual school, heal my marriage, and resume my parents' life and responsibilities by taking their place on the boards and committees they were part of.

After all, I was Super Woman, and I could rest when I was dead. My grief, pain, and issues would just have to be suppressed, I did not have time for any of that nonsense. Tears came in those small private moments alone, like the shower or driving an errand. And grief spilled out of me without my having any control or warning.

Eventually, I ran out of money and had to abandon that idea. The amount of programming that it required on an ongoing basis was greater than my funds. Technology was really new, and only trained people knew how to code. I wasn't one of them.

My coach worked with me to find a different way to build a business that would allow me to create an income in a foreign country to support my family, keep my promises, and, hopefully, keep a small amount of my quickly dwindling savings for the future. I had a running tally of how much longer the savings and inheritance would last.

My parents had made me the sole beneficiary of their estate. If their plan had worked as they planned it, then it would have given me years of financial stability. But they had not planned on all the expenses, the change in the stock market, and how fast that money was being used. I remember one day my mother crying to me shortly before she passed that she was broke. I know the drain of their finances was a major contributing factor to her early passing. My hope was that I could live off it long enough to continue to support my grandmother and our family and build a business until I had my own income. That pressure was heavy, and I did my best to carry it, alone.

My second business venture was based on my mother's love of food, dining, and entertaining that I had gotten from her. In her passing, I had all of her recipes, dinner plans, and organization that she had taught me. She taught me how to pull off a dinner party by being well-planned and organized ahead of time, so it looked easy when the company was there. Nobody ever saw the chaos that was there before their arrival, and she was a hostess who people loved to be in attendance for.

My thought was I could solve the problem of everyday family meals and special occasions by creating meal plans, with itemized step-by-step preparation and grocery lists and honor my mother at the same time.

This new business was to be called What's for Dinner.

It was timely, needed, and fit with my passions. I got to work and dove in as deep as I could while still keeping all the rest of the balls in the air.

Like my parents' plans, life got in the way, and that business never took off, either—For ME.

I have learned that thoughts, ideas, and emotions are physical creations. Just because I put it down didn't mean those ideas died. Someone else picked them up and they became major changes in our world. MeetUP replaced Feast of Friends, and there have been countless businesses that addressed the problem of What's for Dinner.

I know so many people who have heard of new businesses and opportunities and thought, "I had the same thought or plan years ago, why didn't I complete it?" That was the idea that was created, and someone else brought it around. Ideas don't die, they just move to the person who is looking for them. Our universal laws are powerful, and I would, eventually, become an expert, but not for many years.

I had one more option in order to keep my head above water and take care of my grandmother. She was almost 97 now, and while she was still fairly healthy, I knew that she was nearing the end. If I could just hold out long enough for her to live her life in peace, then, yes, I could go about the business of living my own life.

With my parents' passing, I now had access to their files. In the tons of paperwork that I found were the files of my paternal grandmother's estate that had still not been resolved and that my father had been fighting for over 20 years. As the sole beneficiary of my father's estate, if I could get that estate issue resolved, and there could finally be funds distributed to the heirs, then that might buy another 6 months. Those 6 months were like a mirage in the desert, but I was a desperate person. I was hanging on by a thread, and I knew that I was fraying quickly.

When my father passed away, the last hold of his side of the family was breaking. All of the family members that I had held dear to me, were busy living their lives, and I was no longer a part of it. I am guessing that's why the final break came, and I lost that entire side of my family, but I think it had to do with the desperate letters I wrote to the lawyer begging for the estate to be resolved.

I know the lawyer became fed up with me, she kept telling me to hire my own lawyer, but my parents had already spent thousands of dollars over the last 20 years, and I was desperately running out of funds. Paying a lawyer to resolve this estate was just not feasible.

This was my Hail Mary, and I could feel my sanity beginning to slip away.

I often wonder about the expectations people have of others. I am sure that nobody knew the extent of my breaking point, and when you have a tough exterior mask, it could be easy to assume that the person was handling the situation, but I wasn't, and nobody knew because nobody cared to ask.

And with the death of my parents, the last of my family, the last of my happy childhood, the last of my treasured traditions, it was all gone and over. I was stuck between what was and what was happening. The world was moving on, but I wasn't.

And then the final straw hit.

I realized that we had less than 3 months of cash left in the bank. Not only would I not be able to support my immediate family, but now I was putting my grandmother's safety at risk as well. All of these sacrifices would be for nothing if I didn't make a change immediately.

My husband decided that he would return to Canada and return to work. I knew that if he left without me, not only was our marriage 100% over, but now the last of my safety net would be going with him. I knew we "planned" on his working and sending me money, but I now was also wise to "plans" and how they could go their own direction regardless of what I thought or did. I could not control external outcomes.

I made the difficult decision to ask my grandmother to return to Canada with me. If she did that, I could create a separate space for her in my home and still care for her. My husband would be working, we could sell her house, and I could keep all my promises.

I sucked down my pride, and I told her that I was in trouble, that I was running out of money, and that I needed to return to Canada. Would she please come with me? Her reply was no. She would not leave, and could I tell her when her dentist appointment was?

As babies we are unaware of the problems, pressures, and needs of our caretakers, we just demand that our needs be fulfilled. I discovered that was also the case when we were ending our time here. My grandmother had become myopic and could only see what she needed and wanted and was totally unaware of my struggles.

I left that conversation and returned to my place in the house. I yelled at the sky, and at God, and I totally surrendered. I told God that I gave up. I had tried plans A, B, and C and gone all the way to plan E, but nothing I did was working, and I gave up. I tried so hard to keep my promises and my responsibilities. I tried everything that I knew of and more. I was discovering how powerless I was by trying to control and make things happen. I surrendered it all to God, the Universe or Source, or whatever it was.

And then, I fell to my knees and sobbed. I sobbed, curled in the fetal position, sounding like a wounded animal. I sobbed all the grief that I had been suppressing for years. I sobbed out the pain of losing my mother and father, I sobbed about the loss of my marriage and partner that I needed, I sobbed out the loss of my sister, and the loss of my extended family. I sobbed about the failed businesses and how money was so elusive. I sobbed out all of the struggle, pain, loneliness, and isolation that I felt. I sobbed until I was spent.

That was when a miracle happened and I was to get another lesson in the power of the Universe. A woman that I had come to know showed up and invited me to dinner, her treat. She took me to a roadside pizza place that cooked in a wood-fired oven. It was a moment of calm sitting eating pizza in Mexico.

She then asked if she could align my chakras. I had no idea what chakras were at that time, but I had surrendered because I was empty and broken. I went along with it. It felt unusual and foreign, but I played along.

The next day, literally within 24 hours of my breakdown, a solution to all my problems just arrived. A lovely woman and her spouse were looking for a place to live. They would look after my grandmother and do all that I had done for her in exchange for living in the home. I could leave the next week with my husband, we could afford to drive home and still put food on the table while he got a job. My grandmother was taken care of, this lovely couple got a beautiful home to live in, and I could begin to rebuild my life and heal myself. My husband and I could try to heal our failing marriage, and I could try to be the best mother possible to my children.

Why did I think that I had to do it all in the first place? Why didn't I consider this almost 2 years ago? Why did I sell all my belongings, move to a foreign country, and use all my personal savings and inheritance to try to step into someone else's life and their decisions?

I am happy to say that the solution worked out for everyone for another year and a half.

I had to place my grandmother in assisted living at age 98 when she fell and broke her hip. Like many elderly people, a fall tends to coincide directly with a sharp decline, and my grandmother had lost everything that made her who she was.

She lived until she was 102 in the best places I could find. I carried the stress of trying to ensure she was well-cared for long distance in another country, managing her expenses, her health, her decisions, and her quality of life. I had never experienced the true exhaustion of caretaking like that had on me before. I wasn't prepared, but like all the times before, I did my best to soldier on and suppress, suppress, suppress.

My Healing Journey

COVID was many things to many people, but in my perspective, it was a reset button. We were taken out of our routines and our schedules and came face-to-face with ourselves. As a collective, we all had to face some buried truths, and the fallout has been a massive societal paradigm shift.

I talk about this every chance I get when I am speaking, writing, or on my Unlearn the Crap TV show. I believe that our unsustainable societal systems are breaking, everything from our medical systems to educational, governmental, and even financial systems.

We are now in a world that has a digital global currency, we have AI/Robotics and Automations coming in. Our workplaces have been disconnected from a physical location to remote working due to the fast pace of technology that was released during the COVID period. The jobs that we have been trained for are either evolving at a rapid pace, or they are being eliminated altogether.

I believe this is part of the universal laws. The law of Rhythm states that we are in constant cycles and that when we reach the extreme end of one cycle, we are beginning the next new repetitive cycle. Just like the days and nights, the seasons of weather, and every other cycle we live with.

The change of the patriarchal ruling class society that has created a massive unfair division of power and wealth is coming to an end. Women are becoming empowered and uniting, forever ending the division of our community that kept us isolated and disconnected from each other and our true selves.

The Universal law of Compensation shows us that we must be equally compensated for our efforts and contributions, and our win/lose society is coming to an end. We are moving towards a win for the collective. I am not referring to a political practice of socialism or communism, but I believe a new collective is being created. I believe that we are discovering our humanness, our inner power, and our personal gifts. I believe that we are finding that we do, all have a purpose, and our life has meaning. That meaning is based on us living our own life, our own destiny, and no longer in servitude to anything or anyone else.

So with that newfound belief, I understand that I had to finally break. Humpty Dumpty needed to once and for all shatter into a million pieces that prevented me from ever being able to piece the pieces back together again.

I had been too strong for too long.

I needed to have it ALL taken away from me. And that is exactly what happened.

I lost my relationships, my dream home, my job, my health, my wealth, and my identity. I literally lost everything.

And I found myself buried under a lifetime of crap.

I am a Gemini not only by the time and date of my birth but totally and absolutely by my personality. I once read that Geminis were born with a telephone in their ear from a sun sign book.

I really do love to talk.

I am also so unbelievably curious about EVERYTHING. Thank God, for the internet now. It makes looking up things that make me curious so much easier.

But when I was growing up, I needed to read books (and I always bought them because I loved keeping that newfound information all around me). I would take courses, go to retreats, hire coaches, watch documentaries, and go to lectures (I really miss the lectures).

Anything and everything that I wondered about was an absolute requirement that I learn as much about it as I could. I would learn until I was satiated on that topic. Enough to know but not enough to be an expert.

Out of curiosity, one day, I wrote out a list of all the people that I had studied under, and it was over 100 at that time. I am still learning every day now.

I used to say that I knew I was like a cat and that I would die as a result of my curiosity, and I do not see that ever stopping. EVER!

I took that curiosity and continuous learning and applied it to my work and my coaching and developed strong salespeople. You see, I have been in sales my entire life, either as an employee in Sales Management or in direct sales, network marketing, and anything else that caught my attention.

I believe in sales when it is an act of service that we give to others. I can't stand the slimy greedy hard-hitting sales of self-serving. To be good at sales in a serving capacity and living with integrity, I believe it requires a large dose of self-awareness, self-growth, and understanding of the human mind and behaviors. When I removed myself from the equation of serving both my teams and my clients, then it felt pure and clean.

After all, I was raised in a belief system that said we were born to serve others. I became good at serving others, which made me successful in business but not successful in my own personal life. I gave everything that I learned away to others and built up a huge bank of knowledge in my life.

I just never gave it to myself.

I never integrated the knowledge into my true evolution, which is why I believe I broke.

I never put myself on my own list.

That day, I sat on the floor in a total mess and realized that I needed to make a choice. Was I going to live or die? There was no longer the option of an in-between, existing and serving.

I have become well-versed in business development, creation, and efficiency. In one of my previous positions as an employee, I was not only an auditor for ISO 9000, but I was so good at root cause analysis that I was made the auditor of the auditors.

I love the ISO methodology, where you find something that could be improved and then dig into root cause analysis. After that, you develop corrective actions and then create procedures to make it automated.

So, when I decided that I wanted to live, just not the way I had been previously living, I immediately thought of both my business and personal knowledge base. My thinking was if I could get to the root cause of why I was broken, create corrective actions to resolve it, and then apply procedures to create a better new way, then I should be able to heal myself.

It made sense to me because if it worked for business, why wouldn't the concepts work for my own healing journey?

At least, I realized that I had nothing to lose. The doctors had only been able to medicate me and have me end up in a bigger mess and on suicide watch. Truly, I could do a better job at healing; after all, I did have a strong vested interest in my success.

It was called My Life.

I was also gifted with the unique opportunity of having Nothing Left to Lose because I had already lost everything.

I found myself alone, in a new apartment. I had sold my house when my partner and I broke up. I made horrible decisions due to my mental state and lost all the proceeds from the sale. I was on sick leave because of my nervous breakdown and burnout, so I did not have a job to go to. My children were adults and living their own lives. My friends were busy and successful, and life was going on like normal for the world around me. I couldn't exercise or move because both of my knees were shot, and I was waiting for both knees to be replaced by surgery.

I was physically weak and sick from the effects of fibromyalgia. Every single square inch of my body was in constant never-ending pain. My knees were destroyed by osteoarthritis, and I needed both of them replaced. I had gained so much weight from the depression and anxiety but also because of the medication and my lifestyle. I was drinking and eating too much.

I was totally and completely alone with no responsibilities, nobody to answer to, nobody to be involved with.

Just ME.

I had never in my life had that kind of freedom of time, thought, or energy.

I had become a single sole supporting parent at 21. I worked 3 jobs and completed my education while raising my son.

As an employee, I always took on more than was necessary, and to make it look like it was easy for me, I would work free overtime, bring work home, or bring my son to work and work all weekend alone in the office.

I got married at 33 and had my second child at 34. When I was 44, I lost both of my parents 7 weeks apart from each other, which resulted in my being solely responsible for my 94-year-old grandmother, who was living in another country.

I was always entrepreneurial, so in my spare time, I was either working hard to develop an online business or build a direct sales networking marketing business(es).

I believed that I was "supposed" to serve so I was always volunteering for something. I was part of numerous service clubs and, of course, that meant I needed to be on the executive board and add my skills to the club. I am creative and passionate, and that meant that I usually chaired committees or events.

Serving didn't just mean for my community, it also meant for my family and friends. Whenever, and unfortunately, I truly mean whenever, anyone needed anything, I always offered my services. That meant anyone could count on me to help them move, paint, watch their children or pets, clean their house, cook food, and prepare vacations and holidays. I would give anything that I had if anyone needed it, even if I needed it more than they did.

Don't forget my insatiable appetite for continuous learning. I always had something on the go that I was working on, whether it was certifications for an employer, a new skill or talent training (I am a certified interior designer, stock and options trader, plus so many more).

For the very first time in my life, I didn't need to consider what anyone else needed or wanted from me. I was no longer afraid of losing anyone or offending anyone. I had lost everything and everyone, all of my fears had happened, and the miraculous thing was that I was still alive and breathing.

There was profound freedom in that. A freedom that I consider a gift from the Universe from my current perspective but at the time, it was difficult to see it as a gift.

I could sleep as much as I wanted or needed. I could let my body wake up when it was rested. I could eat when I was hungry. I could use the restroom when my body wanted to, not when I had a moment's opening in my day. I could take the time to get in touch with who I was, how I thought and functioned, and really become intimate with myself.

At first, I will admit that I fought it. I kept looking for the answers from outside of myself. I believed people when they told me that they had the solution that I needed and all I had to do was pay them this many thousands of dollars, and my life would be well.

I believed them because I could not believe in myself, yet.

I paid and followed their advice. I did as I was told. I was an overachiever and always did more than was required in less time than was expected.

The value of what I received was priceless. Sorry, that is the wrong word, it was worthless.

All that I got was an empty savings account and deeper in debt. I had more exercises, processes, and strategies than ever, and yet, me and my life were still broken into pieces.

I went to therapy and counseling. I was able to share my lifetime of knowledge and all of these processes with the counselors because, in truth, I was more educated and researched than they were. I was able to teach them so much.

But it did not do ME any good at all, personally.

I moved on to Plan B. I would invest in vitamins, exercise programs, grounding mats, meditations, and alternative healing methods. I sought out acupuncture, massage, homeopathy, salt room therapy, and neuro-linguistic programming. I paid for neurofeedback healing, energy healing, and anything else that I could find.

I left no stone unturned. I left no penny unspent.

I would journal for hours a day.

I pushed myself into building a new network marketing business, thinking that if I just became successful, that might fix all my problems. I am sure it is obvious that was not the solution, especially for someone with a complete nervous breakdown, physically in agony, and unable to walk very far. But at least, that was a strategy that had worked in the past, so I had to give it a try as well.

At least, I could tell myself that I had literally tried everything that was available to me. I truly tried everything that all the "experts" told me to do.

I was left with only one last resort.

I had to go inward. I had to Unlearn my Crap that had taken me so far off course. I had to Unlearn the Crap that I had been told.

I have built a practice of helping my clients uncover and unlearn their crap. Here are some of the foundational beliefs that I use to help people find clarity and direction in the direction of their dreams and purpose that I learned through my life lessons.

If you feel aligned with these words and concepts, I encourage you to reach out and not go it alone. I am here to help you find your path and purpose, so you can live with peace, passion, and prosperity.

We are electromagnetic, biochemical, mechanically interrelated, interconnected energy systems that live within an electromagnetic, biochemical, mechanically interrelated, and interconnected world.

What the hell does that mean?

Aren't we just mere mortal humans? Absolutely NOT.

Aren't we spiritual beings living in a physical world? Yes.

In our lives, we are taught the mechanics of our world and how "things" work. We need these skills to operate all the tools, gadgets, and resources within our homes and workplaces.

Have you learned that you are a mechanical system as well? Your body can easily be equated to a machine. Our heart is like an engine pumping resources throughout the system, our veins are the pipes and tubes delivering fluids, our filtration system is our kidneys and liver, and our coolant system is the lungs and sweat glands. We have a central control system with our brain and nervous system, our digestive system delivers our fuel, and our muscles are hydraulic systems. We have a structural frame with our skeleton and joints and bearings for our movement and flexibility. We have a sensory system that brings information into the entire system.

Do you feel like you are a machine or a car?

It is all so similar. We do not have one set of physical systems for our outer world and a different system for our body. Unfortunately, we have not been taught the basics of how our body operates and how to understand the language of gauges, sending us information constantly.

Our electromagnetic system is the pure energy of our cells. At the cellular level, EVERYTHING is nothing but pure energy and potential. Once activated, that energy can only be transferred or transmuted.

How does our body transfer energy? Through electro pulses like our heartbeat or the synapses of our brain neurons transferring information from cell to cell, it pulses through our nerves and our nervous system.

Have you ever known anyone who has nerve pain? It is the most excruciating pain we know. It feels like you are being electrocuted from the inside out. It feels like that because you literally are. We think of electricity as a source of energy that we capture and use, but energy is energy and we are at the root of all, nothing but pure energy. I know someone who has a rare nerve disorder that they call the suicide disease because the pain is so debilitating.

I said that we were also biochemical systems that were interconnected and interrelated. Have you ever thought about your metabolism other than feeling like a victim of it when it comes to your weight?

Our metabolism is responsible for breaking down and creating chemical reactions within our body. The enzymes in our body are proteins that speed up the biochemical reactions needed for digestion, energy, and so many other functions. The mitochondria in our cells convert glucose and oxygen to feed our cells.

Our DNA is reproduced in full every 7 years by protein reproducing itself, and our hormones are the chemical messengers that regulate our body processes. Our immune system uses biochemical reactions to keep us healthy and ward off disease. Our entire detoxification system keeps our body clean by excreting toxins from our body.

Each of the biochemical systems works together with each other as a complicated system, and when one system is negatively affected, it affects the whole.

Your emotions are chemical responses that vibrate electrically within and outside of your physical body.

Your thoughts are created from chemicals, and they create electromagnetic activity in vibrational waves, and like all vibrational waves, they align with the same vibrations in our world. Like attracts like.

That is our body, our vehicle. Knowledge and communication are your power with your body. I learned that the hard way by just ignoring what I didn't understand or have an answer for. Just like Julia Roberts said in *Pretty Woman:* "Big Mistake. Big Mistake."

The universal laws were always something that I had heard about but really didn't grasp the importance and impact of truly understanding them until I had my breakdown. The universal laws are the equivalent of the rules of the road for driving.

When we understand how the environment around us works, we can easily work with the flow, and when we don't, we can clearly see the consequences. When we drive the wrong way on a one-way street, it makes sense that we can't move easily and there are other cars coming towards us.

When we truly understand all 12 of the universal laws, we can see the signs, navigate with ease, and trust the road. I discuss these in detail in my book **"Unlearn the Crap about Personal Success and Empowerment"**, so for the sake of clarity, I will share a brief understanding of the forces we can navigate when we understand their concepts.

Energy can not be created or destroyed. I learned this important lesson when I took my child on a field trip to a nuclear facility and that was the first thing they said on the tour.

The **Universal Law of Energy** states that everything is energy. Quantum physics has proven that at the very core of EVERYTHING is pure energy. That energy is potent potential until consciousness comes into the equation and then it can become a wave or a particle (energetic vibration or physical manifestation)

The **Universal Law of Oneness** connects the fact that everything is energy by showing us that if at the core of all is the same, there can be no separation. We are made of that which created us. We are creators and we are already connected to the source of abundance. It is only our beliefs and perspectives that give us the illusion of separateness. We do not need to be worthy or earn anything. We are. Period.

Any lack, pain or disconnection is all in our own creation and is part of the crap we need to unlearn.

The **Universal Law of Vibration** explains how we experience the oneness and energy as different aspects because everything vibrates at different rates of speed and frequencies. Everything vibrates and those vibrations align just like a radio station can be picked up by any number of receivers aligned to the frequency of the channel. We can feel the vibrations in our emotions, our senses and in our physical body. Our brain is wired by the frequency of the vibrations and we have the power to change the speed of the vibration though conscious (or unconscious) choice. That is how we can change our reality.

The Universal law of Cause and Effect helps us to understand that everything matters. Every thought, every action, every one, matters and all that we do, say and are creates effects. We can only be victims if we do not see how we are causing our results. I actually do not believe in victims and I know I will cause some resistance with that statement. The reason I shared all my experiences with you is to show you how I was able to see how my beliefs caused me to create what I did not want. Let me clarify here, that does not mean blame. It is about empowerment and when we see and own our own true power, then it is impossible to be a victim. Victor Frankl is a perfect example of how even as a holocaust survivor he understood that he still had the power of his thoughts. When we choose to see ourselves as a victim, we have given away our power.

The **Universal Law of Correspondence** shows us that what is within is equal to what is on the outside. Our reflection in the mirror is equal to the image we present. Our external results are a direct reflection of our inner thoughts, beliefs and feelings. We can not change our results by focusing on results. We must go inward. Our power resides within us and we are more powerful than we know.

The Law of Attraction is the most misunderstood law in my opinion. With so many experts talking about this law from the advent of the movie The Secret we have come to believe that we must change who we are in order to change our results and attract the life we want. That is Crap that must be unlearned. We already are. We know that with the law of Energy and Oneness. We must remove the Crap that is in the way, that is blocking the attraction process if we are not getting our desired results. We live in an abundant universe where we can have it all. Any lack we experience is the result of the crap in the way.

The Law of Action is the part of the Law of Attraction that most people miss out on. You can't just think or feel your dreams into existence. That is only part of the creation process. There must be action. We must align the energy and physical to manifest anything. Let me give an example of this. If we choose to create a baby, we can think we want it, we can imagine and envision, we can have all the affirmations in the world believing it will happen but without sperm connecting to an egg, there is no creation. Action is part of the equation.

The next laws are my favourites. They are my favourites because they show us where our power truly lies. The previous ones were to help us understand the world we live in. This is where we truly create.

The Universal Law of Relativity states that everything exists relative to something else. Which means we are all creating our own realities. There is no absolute truth. Nobody has the same reality as anyone else. Our world is shaped by our beliefs, our thoughts, our filters and our experiences. It is our perception of our reality that we experience. Our eyes do not see. Our ears do not hear. They are receivers of vibration that our brain filters and creates meaning to those vibrations. It is our meaning that creates our reality. If we want a different reality all we need to do is change our perspective and our story.

One of the ways we can do that is with the **Law of Polarity**. Everything has a polar opposite. I know I explained how this understanding was paramount in healing my past and my traumas. If we want to experience love we will have to know the absence of love. That can be experienced with loss or through hatred or evil. We can not banish the side we do not want to experience because trying to banish that which must exist actually gives it more power. We choose to focus our attention on the side we want to experience knowing that the opposite exists. This is where gratitude comes into play. When we know we can choose what we experience, we can be grateful knowing that the opposite is also possible.

This is such an important law for me and one that I work with my clients with all the time. I have seen profound healing taking place by utilizing the power of this knowledge. I have seen how knowing when we are putting our goodness into the world, we will be met with ugly, hatred or evil. When we see it as an inevitable experience of the good we are putting into the world, then we are not being punished or abused by its existence. It just is.

The Universal Law of Compensation states that there MUST be equal compensation for our actions and contributions. This is the law of hope for me. When we focus on our actions and our contributions and leave the results to the universe, we know that we will be compensated equally which means we must focus on what we want our compensation to be and be cognizant of our choices of our contribution. Some people call this the law of Karma.

The Universal Law of Gestation goes hand in hand for me with the Law of Compensation. There is a gestation time for all creation and that time might not be what we want it to be. This is where should's or expectations can take us off course if we believe that our compensation was "supposed" to happen on our perceived or desired timeline. You have heard of Divine Timing, this is it. This is trust that when you have done your part, this is acceptance and surrender. Do not for a moment think that acceptance and surrender are passive or victim traits as we have been taught. That is part of the crap we need to unlearn. We have been made to believe that surrender is for the weak but like vulnerability, it is the true power and strength we possess.

The Universal Law of Rhythm shows us that there is a rhythm and cycle to everything. Understanding where you are in relation to the rhythm makes acceptance and surrender easier. We do not fear the night will last forever as we know that the sun will rise in the morning. We trust that spring will follow the harsh winters and creation will blossom.

We can see the power of the law of rhythm in every aspect of life. There are fractal patterns that are repeated in physics, biology and chemistry. We have mathematical patterns that repeat in fibonacci sequences that create our ability to predict and understand energy, spirituality, astrology, and the unknown.

When we have self knowledge of our own personal alignment with our own rhythms we can work within our natural strengths and creation becomes effortless.

The Universal law of Gender shows us that there is masculine and feminine in everything and everyone. It is the balance and homeostasis of the rhythm of moving within these traits that give us our true empowerment rather than being focused on only one aspect.

Just like when we use the universal laws as a source of information, for critical thinking to make well-thought-out decisions from our choices, so can understanding the archetypes and masks we use become additional information about ourselves.

There are numerous archetypes that we have used for centuries to identify a personality type. We probably have experienced all of them in our lives, but we tend to have some key types that play out in our belief systems. Archetypes are the masks and identities that are universal. The basic archetypes are the caregiver, the hero, the lover, the warrior, the jester, the magician and the orphan.

We use our archetypes to mask our vulnerabilities or to play a part of our expectations. Understanding how our CRAP is played out in archetypes gives us the language of perception. I believe that this self knowledge allows us the clarity to discern if we are in or out of our alignment.

We can't change what we don't acknowledge, and we can't acknowledge what we do not see.

All of these tools are designed to be reflective, feedback systems of information to allow you to navigate and create with ease. But without the knowledge of them, we are at the force of their power without knowing where they come from.

This is designed to pull back the veil and see clearly.

Everybody lives in constant, never-ending, all-over body pain every single moment of the day. Right?

This is normal. I am normal.

Doesn't everybody live on Advil and Tylenol? It sure appears to be normal, especially when I walk down the aisle at the store and see the huge selection of painkillers available. There is a pill for everything.

That was what we were trained to believe. If there is something wrong with you, then you are broken and require outside intervention that usually results in someone else's profits.

For years, I tried to find the reason with my medical team. They sent me on a battery of tests looking for cancers, diseases, or tumors. Every test was looking for the physical issue to be resolved.

I remember about 30 years ago, I came back from one of my tests, and the doctor told me that they didn't find anything but that they saw that I was developing a "fatty liver." When I asked what that meant, I was told it was no big deal, and not to worry about it.

Even then, I thought that did not make sense, but I am older than Google, so what did I know?

I used to be a die-hard smoker. When I was born, my mother was almost late for the delivery room appointment because she wanted to finish her cigarette first. That is how I thought I would spend my life as well.

I remember talking to non-smokers and asking how they lived without smoking. How did they wake up? How did they process their food after eating or how did they manage stress and triggers? And sex?

Until around my late 30s, I was so exhausted and winded that walking upstairs to go to bed was the equivalent of running a marathon for me.

I would get to the top of the stairs and have to spend about 10 minutes slowing my breathing and heart rate down enough to get to bed.

I thought the issue was smoking, and when I was desperate enough to quit and give up my best friend. I did.

At that moment, I realized the power of decision and identity. For a die-hard smoker to just quit without issues, it was like a miracle to learn the power of a decision.

I have never smoked again.

But I was still exhausted and winded.

So, I quit my morning coffee, thinking it was caffeine.

Nope. Still couldn't make it up the stairs.

Here I was in my 30s, "supposedly" the most powerful time of my life physically, and I had to work up the energy and courage to walk up the stairs to go to bed.

I realized that I had done everything that I could think of, I had tried Plans from A to G, and still moving around in my home was utterly and totally exhausting.

So, I did what I always did, when I couldn't find the answer myself, I turned outside of myself to the "experts," and I went to the medical community.

After a battery of blood work, I was "diagnosed" with Hyperthyroidism. Does that make any sense to you? It did not to me, either. How could I be so exhausted that I had to take multiple naps during the day and still struggle with the marathon of the nightly stairs?

But what did I know? I wasn't a doctor, so even though it felt totally wrong and counterintuitive, I took the thyroid pills.

And the pills worked. They took away my hyperthyroidism and gave me hypothyroidism.

That was my first memory of becoming a living experiment for Big Pharma.

Every month, I had to go to the doctor, get blood work, and see where my TH levels were. Back then, your results were kept a secret, and I was only told the interpretation of the results by the "expert" doctors.

I remember the first time I saw actual medical test results. I was in Mexico while my father was in his transition stage (nice way of saying he was dying) from complications of alcohol abuse. He had developed type 2 diabetes, which developed into renal failure. The doctor gave me my father's lab results, and I was shocked. "You mean I am 'allowed' to know the results and actually see them?" When I read the results, even though they were in Spanish, I understood them immediately.

Do you know that lab results show you the range of normal beside the results?

I realized that was part of the "control and power" we had given away about our health. That was 16 years ago as I write this.

I felt controlled by the pills just the same way that I felt controlled by cigarettes, and I did not like it all. I was determined to get myself off the pills even though I had been told that now that I was on them, this was a lifetime commitment.

I now know that is the purpose of medication—keeping lifelong built-in customers. Medication is not for healing the root cause.

It was in the early 2000s, and I was becoming exposed to alternative health modalities. The Universe brought me answers even when I wasn't actively looking. (Another theme that I was being exposed to but never really explored its power until I had my breakdown.)

I was introduced to a woman who could connect through the energy of my body through a sample of my hair.

The process involved putting a piece of my hair into her machine and letting the energy of the universe heal what my body wanted to be healed. It felt like voodoo or magic at the time, and my doctor called it quackery, but when it healed what was setting my thyroid off-kilter, the results could not be denied.

I told the doctor that I had stopped taking my medications, and he was appalled. I remember thinking that it felt like I was being chastised by a parent or teacher for doing something without their prior permission.

But it was MY BODY and MY LIFE, and I knew instinctively that pills were not the answer.

When my blood work came back saying that I was normal and I felt like myself again, the doctor told me that he did not believe in what I was doing, but it was working, and as long as I agreed to do monthly blood work to keep an eye on it, then he would support my decision. After 6 months of blood work tests, he told me to keep doing what I was doing.

"Future medicine will be medicine of frequencies"
—Albert Einstein

Does it make you question why our society follows Einstein on so many things that make a profit, but when it defies the current profit centers, it is ignored? It sure does for me.

Since that first initiation into energy healing I have explored so many options. It was my go-to when I had my complete breakdown and felt like I lost my mind. I do not believe in coincidences, so when I had an ad hit my social media feed (yes, I know algorithms brought it to me, and that is part of the evolution we are in), I followed up immediately with a process for brain healing called Neuroptimal. It is a machine that uses binary sounds to activate the brain, thereby creating feedback to the brain. Our unconscious mind needs feedback in order to see what is there, otherwise it is on autopilot.

As I sat in the comfortable chair, listening to music and relaxing, my brain was pulsing and working to reset all the damage that my life had done to it. It took about 10 sessions, and I went from sobbing at every appointment to beginning to smile and talk normally again.

In my opinion, everything needs a mirror or some kind of feedback system in order to see clearly, which is why I now challenge as much of my own thinking, beliefs, and habits as possible.

We can not fix or heal what we do not acknowledge. And we can't acknowledge what we are unaware of.

Conscious awareness has become a core value of all that I do and share. It is through our own consciousness that we have the ability to make informed decisions through the choices we make.

Even though I know and believe that, I still struggled when it came to my own health.

I was so impressed with the process that I became a certified practitioner for Neuroptimal, and I highly recommend it. The thing that I really love about energy healing is that we do not need to be retraumatized in order to heal trauma. We can let our body release it and just let it go.

For me, talk therapy felt like re-entering the battlefield each time. Yes, I became a bit numb to the battlefield the way I think soldiers become battle fatigued, but it never healed the root cause. It never let me go and become free from it.

I had spent a lifetime learning to "live with" my trauma. It was slowly eating away at my soul and my zest for life. I wanted HEALING, not management.

Unfortunately, the Western medical system is based on drug therapy, medical procedures, and pain management. We do not go into healing the root cause. It is almost like each trauma, each pain, means we are victims, and we are stuck with the results we have.

That just never ever made sense to me. Now that I am really understanding and living with the universal laws, I know it is totally against the natural laws. If we do not like the effects, we must address the cause.

That is the law of Cause and Effect with our personal power.

The Law of Compensation has taught me that we will be equally compensated for our contributions and efforts, regardless of whether they are empowering or disempowering. I was equally compensated for ignoring my body signals and pleas for help and attention with a lot of pain and disease.

I wish my story of how I learned to take control of my own health ended here, but the "Crap" that I had been taught was so ingrained that when the crisis of the moment relented, I fell back into old habits and beliefs.

When I was almost at rock bottom, I remember my current doctor truly trying to figure things out for me. I was EXHAUSTED. I couldn't sleep, I was in constant pain, and I was barely holding on.

I blamed my inability to sleep on my mattresses and pillows. I purchased mattress after mattress. I bought 6 different mattresses over the course of 8 years. I bought every pillow that existed, from water pillows, bean pillows, foam, etc. I truly spent tens of thousands of dollars on products trying to get a night's sleep.

Every morning the alarm clock went off, and I could quickly calculate how much time it took to get things done in order to leave for work, and I would snooze until the last possible second.

Then, with coffee and Diet Coke, I would push through the day. When the pain hit, I always had my over-the-counter pain meds there, and together, they would push me through the day.

My doctor asked if I had trauma. NO. Don't be ridiculous, that didn't happen to me. Sure, I had been verbally, emotionally, physically, and sexually abused, but I had that under control, and it was in the past, so it didn't count. I truly discounted everything that I had endured because that was how I coped.

My doctor put me on antidepressants and sleep aids.

That didn't fix anything. It did make me less aware of what my body was trying to tell me, but that was all.

My big aha moment was when I went to a skilled masseuse. She told me that there was no way I should be in the amount of pain I was experiencing by her touching me. This was not normal. She believed that I had fibromyalgia and wanted me to get tested before she would even agree to have me on her table again. Talk about integrity. Nobody had ever been like that with me before.

Google now existed, so I could do a deep dive into the condition. OMG, there was a name for what I was experiencing, and I told my doctor. I think he was finally relieved that he could do something for me because he truly was and is an amazing person and kind man.

We began the experimentation of drugs again, not strong enough, too strong, until we felt we had found the just right place. I realized that for the first time in my life, I was living without the experience of constant, never-ending, all-over body pain. I had to be on a large mix of drugs to get there, but this was what "normal" felt like.

My doctor asked me if I felt we had the right mix, and I couldn't answer him. I asked him to describe what "normal" people felt, I was that disconnected from my own body.

But the medications, when added to no other life changes, just masked the problems. It pushed me to my breaking point but hid the fact that it was coming. I lived with a false sense of security that the medication was making everything ok.

My breakdown was the greatest thing that ever happened to me.

It was the hardest, most painful, most terrifying time of my life. But it was the tie that, when it broke, it set me free.

I have since learned that I was denied the knowledge of how my body works, physically, chemically, and biologically.

As human beings, we are interconnected, interrelated systems. We are electromagnetic, bio-chemical, and mechanical energy systems. Everything is connected to everything. From what we eat, to what we think and what we do, it is all part of the intricate systems of our bodies.

Our central nervous system is our core that is designed to keep us alive. It is a basic on-off switch, and while the 'on' switch is wired with a hair trigger from our ancestors, we can control the 'off' switch.

When we do not turn off our sympathetically activated nervous system, we are living with constant stress. Stress is released from our glands, affects our organs, and how everything works together.

Our emotions are the gauge system that tells us what is happening inside our body. When we suppress our emotions or feel they are out of control, it is equivalent to telling the thermometer it is overreacting when the temperature is high. It is information. We need to use it.

When we do not understand and connect with our body systems, we create illness in our body. Our body's illness can be found in our mental, physical, and emotional states.

If we do not get to the root cause here at this point, the wear and tear creates disease in our body, mind, and soul.

We learn how to operate every piece of machinery in our world, from the car we drive to the machinery we use in our work and everything in between. Our body is a complicated machine or an automation system. If we are using our body without the knowledge of how it operates, we are basically destroying it while thinking there is something wrong with IT!

We would never drive our prized dream car without knowing how to drive. That is the same as crashing and banging into everything, destroying the vehicle while we figure it out, through trial and error.

If our society requires that we have "licenses" in order to legally operate any piece of machinery, we need certifications to use some for our jobs, then how can we be sent out into the world, in the MOST complicated, interconnected, automation system of our physical body, without the basic knowledge of how it works?

It is time that it becomes common knowledge that:

- Our brain is a wired system that gets its information from our senses.
- With that information, our brain creates programs based on what worked for us, and without feedback, our brain believes that if we are still alive, then whatever happened, worked, and it WILL keep repeating the program and pattern.

- We have 3 intellectual centers in our body; brain, heart, and gut. Each with its own responsibilities and capabilities.
- Our emotions are chemically created and electromagnetically transmitted.
- Stress is created when any of these systems are not working properly. It creates friction, and friction creates inflammation.
- Inflammation is the root cause of all diseases.

When we truly know and understand each of our body systems, we can drive our body like we drive a car. We know the warning signs, the sounds of friction, and the feeling of misalignment. We respect and honor that everything our body is providing us is feedback and information. We can correct and continue, with the most subtle cues when we know how to listen to them.

We are powerful beyond our imagination when we are not fighting our own bodies.

I am so thrilled to know that medical science is finally understanding that we are whole complete beings and we can't be dissected into pieces. The medical community is now leading trials about the connection of the mind and body, to stress and inflammation and how physical, emotional, and mental health are all intertwined.

They understand that chronic stress is the root cause of autoimmune diseases as well as so many other conditions. Our body, under a constant barrage of cortisol and adrenaline, will begin to fry itself. I know of people who have nerve pain issues, inability to control their own muscles, Parkinson's, and in my case, fibromyalgia. They are learning, and hopefully, soon, we can Unlearn the Crap of a pill for everything and get to the root cause of disease—stress.

And stress comes in so many forms for our body. Stress of malnutrition from our food source, stress from a lifestyle of job, family, keeping up with the "Joneses", excessive consumerism, debt, and so much more. Stress comes from coping mechanisms that develop into addictions. Stress from self-denial, self-sabotage, and self-disrespect, I believe are the true evils. When we are at war with ourselves, we are in constant, never-ending battles.

How can we achieve passion, purpose, peace, and prosperity under those conditions?

* * * *

I don't know why I thought our education system was built on learning and personal development because it truly isn't. I know that is the crap that we have been taught, or indoctrinated into believing, but it is not true.

Our education system was built to create workers for jobs.

Jobs were created by the standardization of the industrial revolution.

The industrial revolution was created for greater profits and efficiencies.

I talked about the history of our education system in my book *Unlearn the Crap about Personal Success and Empowerment,* from how it changed from knowledge access being denied to the majority to keeping the power and control to the few.

When I was going to school, there were so many aspects that I found confusing. Why did some things come so easy to me and make me believe that I was smart and some things were so hard and overwhelming and make me think badly of myself?

I felt like I was "supposed" to be good at everything.

There were scoreboards in the school that showed who had the best overall grades. I was never on that board. I had exceptional grades in languages, arts, and psychology and really bad grades in history, math, and science (and forget physical education). My physical body was never my strength, and the more stress I put on myself, the faster my body performed even worse.

When my son was born, I sucked up my pride and went on social assistance and returned to school. I began college as a mature student and a young single mother. I was surrounded by young adults having the time of their lives, and I was overwhelmed with responsibility and the joy of learning.

I remember excelling at all my classes, but I just could not comprehend accounting. It was required for me to get my diploma, and this was before the days of computer programs, so I needed to understand the logic of debits and credits, and how you could credit a debit account and vice versa.

It was pure mumble jumble to me, and I felt like a fool. I knew I was smart, and I learned quickly, so why could I not figure this out?

When I thought I finally got it, I remember taking my assignment to the teacher proud that I had finally conquered this mountain. His response was... WRONG.

I questioned him, why was it wrong, how was it wrong, please help me understand. He told me to go figure it out. It took me taking that course 3 times before I finally got the basis enough to just scrape a passing grade by.

What a waste of my time and energy.

Imagine if I had learned what my core genius was and became an expert in it. Why did I need to be a generalist on everything? But that was how our school system worked.

I read a book called the *Outliers* by Malcolm Gladwell. The book is all about his research into what makes some people extraordinarily successful and others not. There was a story in there that has forever stuck with me.

He talked about the amount of artists that the Renaissance period created. It seems that once a child was recognized as being artistic, they would be sent away to live and be mentored by an artist. That child was then raised in an environment that not only supported their inner genius but also nurtured it and grew it.

Can you imagine if we were all raised in our own genius environment and nurtured to be authentically aligned with ourselves?

I recently have been introduced to a newish study called Human Design. It is a combination of 4 of the ancient studies about how we are and how the energies of our birth created our natural states.

The Human Design System is like a guide that combines astrology, the I Ching, the Kabbalah, and the Hindu-Brahmin chakra system with quantum physics. It helps you see your unique energetic blueprint, making it easier to understand your strengths, challenges, and purpose. There are five types: Manifestors, Generators, Projectors, Reflectors, and Manifesting Generators. Each type has its own way of making decisions and experiencing life, helping you on your path to self-discovery and living authentically.

I discovered that I am a Manifestor.

A Manifestor is about 10% of the population and we are designed to initiate and create. I need to be constantly learning and then sharing that knowledge.

That explains so much about who I am, how I feel my best, and why I have "failed" at so many things. I failed at the things that I was trying to push on myself because of "supposed to" or "shoulds". Not because it was who I was.

I try to imagine how my life would have been different if my parents had known about Human Design. Who would I be now, if I had learned these lessons earlier in my life rather than as a result of a breakdown?

Creating my source of income and how I spend my time, along with my natural strengths rather than the evolution of society and my past has made all the difference in my mental and physical health.

I encourage you to learn as much as can about yourself. When you become an expert in you, and then make choices that are aligned with you, now you are empowered.

I recently had a conversation while being interviewed for a PBS show called *Recipe for Wellness* by Sanjay Raja. We were discussing the need to be pushed to our limits in order to build resiliency. I challenged him on that topic, and I can't stop thinking about that concept.

What if we were taught who we were authentically, how our body worked to know intrinsically if we were aligned internally and externally with our authentic selves and knew of the universal laws and how they worked. Could we use that knowledge to handle our own challenges, self-direct ourselves, and build resiliency from the inside out?

I believe we could.

We are always more committed to change when it is our mission, our purpose and we have something important to guide us. Learning resilience from a place of external force tells me that we are still living in unproductive, unhealthy stress.

Stress is used as a power source to fuel our lives, our dreams, our intentions, our goals, and our true life, now, isn't that what a true fuel source is to be used for?

I have been listening to a neuroscience podcast by Andrew Huberman called the Huberman Lab Podcast. In one episode, he was talking about the different ways our brain learns. We first learn by situational, that is, our brain takes in our environment and our events and creates neural pathways of beliefs, learning, and adaptability with it. It is automatic, and our brain is doing its own wiring. That process lasts from birth up until about age 25.

After age 25, our brain learns by self-directed learning. We choose what we want to learn. We create focus and attention. We learn something, and when we go to sleep, our brain does the wiring process and cements it in.

We learn by removing what doesn't work through practice. That means we all begin through failure. Failure is the starting point. It is not a judgment or a life sentence. With enough practice, both physically, mentally, and through visualization, we can wire our own brains from ineptitude to expertise. It is a choice. It is a practice.

Again my question comes up with, what if our education system was based on the individual?

What if we first learned who we were by being exposed to many stimuli, learning if we are emotional, physical, or intellectual learners? Learning all about ourselves intimately?

Add in knowing our energetic blueprint with whatever energy modality works for you, personally, I love the blend that Human Design gives, and I am actively studying it myself.

Then, add in the universal laws of how our external world functions, combine all of that, and then choose our mission and purpose based on who we are. Then, add in the passive and self-directed learning, and become more of ourselves every day.

What if we all were living in complete and total alignment with who each of us was, and together, we weaved a fabric of individuality, creating an overall canvas of life?

Would there be any problem that we could not solve in our world? Would our oceans, our trees, and our environment be in jeopardy? Would anyone go without basic needs? Would we need to fight and have wars if we were all a part of the whole, living our individual best lives?

Sounds like utopia in our current world state, but isn't that the world we used to live in before control and power of domain were forced on us?

* * * *

It didn't seem to matter where I went, strangers would just start telling me their intimate personal problems, and I was always able to come up with solutions. Most of those solutions involved my own self-sacrificing.

The biggest crap that I needed to Unlearn was that others were more important than me, that I needed to put other's needs before my own.

That crap took me down and almost out.

Which "others" I never was able to identify, so that meant everyone else. How does one person serve everyone else when they all have different needs?

Did it mean only my intimate family or my extended family? What about employers and coworkers? Or my community?

How was I to serve all of them before myself? And most importantly, who then served me?

These are questions that I wished I had stopped long enough to ask myself rather than just working so hard to fulfill this illusion that my role was to take care of the world.

Let's start with this thought. Who the hell am I that I am so omnipotent that I have the power and capacity to take care of the world?

How did I even come to this conclusion? As I took inventory of my thoughts, actions, and beliefs, it came from so many sources. It came from the polite rules of etiquette of being a host and social conformities.

It came from 'what happens at home, stays at home.'

Never let anyone see you cry.

Put on your big girl panties and get to work.

You can sleep when you are dead.

It came from being told that I should never let a guest be the last one eating as it made them uncomfortable, so I had to eat past the last person eating. Yet, I wasn't supposed to have an unhealthy relationship with food and hold a healthy body weight.

I don't remember being born and then being told, "Okay, hurry up and grow up so you can take the responsibility from others and carry it yourself."

Part of my healing journey came from becoming an energy healer and learning that our cells and DNA hold the pain of previous generations. That made me think about the women that came before me. Did I inherit these thoughts and beliefs?

My maternal grandmother was born in Estonia in 1914, and she lived until 102. She was strong and independent, and she loved us, her family, so deeply.

Yet she was also so picky and demanding, wanting everything to be perfect. She would pick up every single tomato in the store display to choose only the best one. She did that for every single decision and choice she made in her life. Presents were to be admired and enjoyed and savored rather than rushing to open them. Each piece of wrapping paper was inextricably sliced through the tape in order to preserve every single piece of paper to be reused the next year.

Although it became a source of laughter as we gave her presents every year, I now know that there was a belief or a trauma behind those traits of hers.

She was the youngest child of 5, and her family had very little money. When she was 7 years old, she was "sent to the country" to watch the cows for a farmer. I don't know if her work provided an income to her family or just relief from having to feed her during those summer months, but it was very traumatic for her. Every morning she would have to walk the herd of cows out to a field to graze and then, when evening came, walk them back to the barn. She would be out in the fields all day, alone.

She told me two stories repeatedly, which I now know is a sign of unhealed trauma. The first was she once fell asleep in the field with the cows and did not bring the herd back in time. When the farmer came out to find her, she was severely chastised for failing at her duties. The second story was that when the end of summer arrived, and it was time for her to return to her family and back to school, she was informed that she needed to stay and continue to work for a few more months.

Imagine a 7-year-old child being able to process that. What beliefs did she carry that forever stayed with her? Did she always have to be perfect in order to survive and be accepted? Did she feel rejected or banished and sent away? How could she have a trusting relationship with anyone as an adult if that was wired into her brain?

From my perspective, it made it impossible.

She once told me a story of falling head over heels with a "beautiful boy". He swept her off her feet. The rest of her love story didn't end well. If I understood her cryptic storytelling, I believe she found herself pregnant and rejected. I know she did not have a child at that time, so I can only imagine how she managed that situation back in the 1930s, but it was also the beginning of the Soviet Army taking away the country's independence in June 1940. What a clash of events that she had to endure.

She told me about going to the theater during World War II, which was a big event. Everyone dressed up in their absolute finest clothes and set out for the evening. While the country was under Russian control and the war fought on, she tried to live a "normal" life. While she was at the theater, the building was bombed with everyone inside. She had to run to the safety of the basement bomb shelter and then, when it was over, navigate the destroyed streets in order to get home.

I can't imagine what that experience would do to the feeling of safety that we all crave and how it would forever affect her and us who came from her, but I do know that fear was forever built into her DNA.

She tried to learn to drive and get her driver's license, but when the car felt out of control for her, rather than fighting to keep control of the car, she lifted her hands off the wheel and covered her face. She never ever tried to drive a car again.

Near the end of the war, when Germany was coming and taking over her country and beating the Russians out, she had an opportunity to escape. She and some of her friends found a boat that they could take and leave the country in the dark of night cover. One of the people was brought into the boat because he was a seasoned captain and could navigate the dangerous Baltic Sea, getting them safely to Sweden and a new life.

As they were sneaking onto the boat, they were spotted by some German soldiers, and the terror that shot through her came through when she shared that story. Their escape could easily be taken away, but more than that, they could be captured by the enemy and imprisoned. This was not something that my grandmother was built for. But luckily, the soldiers were just as war-torn as her party was, and then just nodded and turned their heads.

While they were off in the middle of the sea, a huge storm came and knocked that small boat around. Everyone in the boat looked to the seasoned captain, hoping that he had the skills to get them to Sweden safely, but unfortunately, in his own desperation, he had lied to them. He had no knowledge of boats or sailing. He was just as confused and overwhelmed as they were.

When the storm ended, and they saw the land, they were again terrified. None of them knew which country they were headed towards because the storm had them spinning in circles. They knew if they arrived back in Estonia, they would immediately be arrested as prisoners of war. After everything that they had endured to find this escape, enduring the voyage only to have it end in failure was beyond heartbreaking.

She told me the joy that they all felt when they saw a Swedish flag on the land. Their cries of freedom were added to their shredding and tossing of their "official papers" overboard. Their final act of rebellion before landing in a new country and beginning their new life.

My grandmother began her new life in Sweden with her husband and found that she was pregnant with my mother. Everything was about to change for everyone because it appeared that my grandmother's luck in love was continuing. Her husband was having an affair and left her alone and pregnant to begin a life with his new love.

She had a difficult pregnancy, and being alone and broke didn't make things easier. One day after a walk, she came home to her apartment to find her belongings out on the street. It appeared that her husband left her, he no longer felt the need to pay her bills, and she was now alone, pregnant, penniless, and homeless.

When it came time to give birth, she had to be taken to a "bad women's" hospital because she was deemed a single mother. She was taken to the hospital on the arms of a bicycle because that was all that was available to her. She carried the shame of being alone, rejected, broke, and now a mother with the strength that I can only imagine.

Throughout my grandmother's long life, she never remarried, never lived with anyone, and remained fiercely independent. She made money stretch farther than anyone I have ever met and always had more than many in my life. She managed her money and her life from a place of fear of losing independence. She did so from a place of a low-paying job and not ever being taken care of by anyone.

As I look at her story and my life, I have to ask myself some deep questions. Why did I feel that I needed to serve others before myself? Did her demands of perfection and independence translate to me being of service? What effects did her story have on my mother, which were then passed on to me?

My father fell immediately, head over heels, in love with my mother at first sight. Literally.

He was a teenager coming into his own when he spotted a young beautiful girl across the street. Immediately captivated by her, he asked his friend, "Who is THAT?" His friend replied, "That? That's just Lena." My father immediately told his friend, "That is not Just Lena, that is the woman I am going to marry."

And he did.

Earlier than anyone expected. My parents were becoming teenage parents, and without any other option, my father insisted that my mother marry him. She did, and they remained together for the rest of their lives. But they did it at a cost to both of them. While they loved each other deeply, the cost came at the expense of their individual dreams and goals.

My parents passed away too young, 7 weeks apart, and I became the matriarch of the family in my 40s and was responsible for my 94-year-old grandmother in another country.

From the outside, my mother had achieved the "American dream". She had a fantastic career, rose the corporate ladder, and had a middle-class home, friends, and a fantastic social life. She traveled the world with my father and retired early to Mexico with my father and her mother.

And yet she died before she turned 60, with a life of regrets of what she could have done or could have been. She KNEW she had more in her and felt that she had thrown it away by her choices as a teenager.

For me, I grew up always knowing this story of how I came to be and how it affected my mother. I always knew that if she had the option of terminating her pregnancy, she would have. She knew that being a teenage mother and bride were not the expectations of her from her family. She knew she was destined for more, she was intelligent, passionate, and creative. She was special, and everyone around her knew it. She was magnetic, and she was my hero.

I know that I had turned that knowledge into a belief that I did not belong here and that I needed to earn my right to be. It was the foundational belief that drove me to people pleasing, over-delivering, self-sacrifice, and putting everything and everyone ahead of myself.

It's funny, though, because I could never have told you that was my belief. I couldn't articulate it or identify it while I was too busy living it. It just was my reality.

It was only when I began my healing journey and challenged my behaviors, my thoughts, my results, and looked at root cause analysis that I was able to see it clearly.

I believe that is the power of limiting beliefs, in the dark, they thrive like a parasite and drive our unconscious choices, but in the light of challenge, it becomes crystal clear that they do not even make sense.

In hindsight, I can see the breadcrumbs of my grandmother's trauma creating beliefs of fear of rejection, fear of failure, and the need to be perfect and how that affected how she raised my mother.

My mom had this standing joke that she was so perfect that she didn't even have bodily functions. We used to work hard to catch her passing gas, and she would deny it strongly. I thought it was just a joke.

But my brain didn't.

I had so many digestive issues all of my life. I suffered from IBS, intense and uncontrollable gas, weight gain, and inflammation. I was unable to go to the bathroom in public, or a gas station, and do not even mention a porta potty. I learned to hold my bodily functions in so much that it was beyond unhealthy. I drank as little water as possible, so I wouldn't have to use the restroom. If there was even a chance that someone would be around me when I needed to have a bowel movement, then I was unable to let go.

I suffered for so many years. The doctors gave me every kind of invasive test, looking for the disease or tumor that was causing my digestive issues. Nobody could find the cause, so I just suffered, which created more inflammation and stress, and my body just kept breaking down.

When I dug into my beliefs during my healing, I realized how this very joke of my mother's had been interrupted by my brain. There was something wrong with me if I had bodily functions, and I must learn to eliminate them at all costs. When it was uncontrollable and I failed, then the shame of my imperfection must be hidden at all costs.

When I challenged my beliefs and thoughts and found this was rooted in a joke, it was impossible to continue to believe it. It is just crazy to think the very life force of digestion is a sign of being unacceptable and imperfect. It is the very process of all life, digesting what is needed, and eliminating what is not.

I am happy to say that as soon as I saw the truth, I did not need anything else to change my belief. It just made immediate sense, and now, I honor my body processes and am thrilled when it is working efficiently. I watch for signs that my digestion is telling me and am developing a profound respect for how well my body has worked, even against my fighting against it.

Unfortunately, my body did not heal as fast as my belief changed. There is a lifetime of damage that I have done, and finding my natural balance is a priority in my journey.

Did my grandmother's need for perfection out of fear of survival make my mother feel the need to measure up and be perfect for her mother? Did that declaration of perfection in her joke show up as a wound for her, and was she overcompensating for not being perfect?

* * * *

Why do we bring the messiness of relationships into our lives?

Besides the fact that it is written in our DNA, that we are social beings. Our survival and ability to thrive are coded right into our cells based on relationships. Failure to Thrive is a disease created from lack of touch, lack of emotions, and lack of connections. Isolation and rejection are the biggest kryptonite that can take us down.

Besides knowing that our hormones and biochemical balance are based on creating dopamine, serotonin, oxytocin, estrogen, and testosterone. Take these hormones out of balance and our ability to function gets increasingly decreased. The lack of these hormones can change our thoughts, our beliefs, and our habits. The lack of dopamine and serotonin creates addictions.

Besides that, there is safety in numbers, and when we are a community, collaborating we increase the success of each other.

Besides all the electromagnetic, socioeconomic, and health reasons... There is one I have taken extremely personally.

Relationships are our mirror.

We see ourselves through other people. It creates our filters, which decide what information gets in and what is repelled from us. It creates our reality and our life.

When I went into relationships with fear of rejection, I always created more rejection. No matter how much I would tell people that they were creating this feeling inside of me and they should change their behavior, I still received more rejection.

When I sought comfort and security from the people in my life, I dragged them down to my level if they let it happen, and I was left feeling unsafe and scared.

When I had my breakdown, I lost everything and everyone.

Every fear I had—happened. Every person I sacrificed myself for, left.

I learned that we can only create from the inside, and yet, we were taught to seek it from external sources. That is part of the crap that needs to be unlearned. I truly believed that I needed to give in order to receive. People pleasing and self-sacrificing are all signs of misalignment.

Lessons I Learned from
Unlearning My Crap

1. We must heal our pain and trauma in the same environment that created the wound.

   The best way to heal is in the moment and where the trauma occurred. But we can only do this from a place of self awareness.

   We will continue to attract our crap until we heal or remove it so when we see cycles and patterns repeating in our lives we need to discern if the pattern is empowering or disempowering.

   If it is empowering for us, then let it be your autopilot but stay aware. We are always changing and evolving and chances are that even the best programming becomes outdated and obsolete.

2. Love is our super power.

   It is a choice, an action and a verb. It is not a feeling that comes and goes. Love will always keep you safe. Love will always be the right choice.

3. We do not make mistakes. We are always doing the best we can.

   And so is everyone else. When we know better, we do better - love this quote from Maya Angelou. If we aren't getting our desired results then we have crap in the way that must be addressed and removed and refer to #1.

4. Triggers are not your weakness. They are the language of your soul.

   Triggers are like champagne bubbles. They have been bottled up and suppressed to such a powerful degree that it requires a wire cage to hold the pressure in. When you are ready to release the pressure, the bubbles burst to the top to be released.

That is what a trigger is.

It is your body, your unconscious mind telling you that you have something that has been suppressed that is ready to be released. Allow it to process through you. Acknowledge to yourself that you have been carrying this burden and set it free. It and YOU are ready to let it go.

5. The very things that are holding you back are the same things you need to propel you to your dream life.

    Our zone of genius resides in the polar opposite of your challenges, traumas, and pains. If you think about the opposites as having a sum total of 100%, then addressing your challenges reduces their weight and adds to your strengths.

    Our challenges are there to point to the direction of our genius. Just turn around and look in the opposite direction, you will see your gifts, your passions, your mission, your vision, your power. Embrace it.

    And each time you are ready to strengthen your zone of genius, those same challenges will appear, but they will be easier to resolve each and every time. Just like grade school was challenging when you were 5 years old, but those challenges are easy when you are in college.

6. Become comfortable with discomfort. That is where the greatest gifts come from.

    Our brains are wired to keep us safe and alive. Not happy. Not healthy. Not wealthy. Alive. If you are comfortable, you are going to stay exactly where you are, getting exactly what you have. If you want anything different, you MUST be uncomfortable.

The beauty is that when you take action in your discomfort, you signal the brain to release the endorphins and chemicals that reward you for your action in order to get you to the next safe place.

7. Words are Not Sticks and Stones. They are your power supply.

    Thoughts are formed by our words. Our thoughts create our emotions and the energy that we omit and attract. Our thoughts create our biochemistry that changes our health and stress responses. Our thoughts and words are the creative force that creates our results. If you don't like your results, change your thoughts and words.

8. Judging anything or anyone else is our soul showing us a mirror about ourselves.

    When we have a strong reaction to something outside of ourselves it is always a mirror about our internal state.

    Pay attention to your strong emotions and feelings. That is your soul's language showing you what needs to be addressed.

    Everything in our experience is only about us. It is the universal laws at full play for our benefit. Every single person is experiencing a different reality and different truth. Everything we experience is processed through our filters of perception. As we unlearn our crap, we expand our capacity to see other perspectives and other realities.

9. Failure is NOT a failure. It is how the brain learns. It must unlearn what is not working in order to learn what does.

    Embrace your failures. Seek to get as many as possible because it is finding and removing what doesn't work that allows you to find what does. It is like Michelangelo carving the statue of David—he had to remove what wasn't David in order to release the essence from the stone.

The only way to fail is to quit.

10. Ignorance is NOT bliss, it's disempowerment.

    Self-awareness is BLISS. Knowing yourself is your greatest source of empowerment. When we ignore, hide, suppress, and avoid, we are giving our power away.

    Knowing your past and acknowledging everything that you have gone through is honoring yourself and your journey. Every part of it is information for your self-awareness.

    Knowing your present and seeing clearly the results you have created (and YES, you have created it all, even if it is unconscious or ancestral, you created it). Once you own the responsibility, you now own the source of your power, and that is something nobody can take away from you.

11. Finding the POSITIVE in everything is not the Law of Attraction.

    The Law of Attraction is based on your vibration and your energy, which originates from your feelings and begins in your thoughts and beliefs.

    Seeing the situation and then CHOOSING which direction to focus on is how you utilize the Law of Attraction. It is simple, but it is not easy. Sometimes, it takes choosing the direction every single second until you have turned the ship around.

12. Happiness is not found in the absence of problems.

    Happiness is an emotion, and emotions are part of the Law of Rhythm. They ebb and flow. Your emotions are meant to keep you in neutral, so if you are experiencing too much outside of your baseline, you will experience the opposite emotion in order to create balance. Consider every time you have heard laughter at a funeral. Your nervous system can't be in extremes for too long.

Enjoy the happiness when it comes. Register it to your brain, knowing it won't last, but it will return.

What does last is purpose and peace.

When you are at peace with your true purpose, you will feel satisfaction and true empowerment. You raise your baseline every time you heal and release a trauma. That is the power, raising your baseline higher and higher, so you become stronger and stronger.

13. Time does not heal all wounds.

Our wounds are part of our story. We can't live a life without experiencing traumas, pains, and wounds. People will leave us, they will die, they will hurt us. We will not have all of our needs met. We will misinterpret situations and create stories that will dictate our belief patterns, and we will retraumatize ourselves.

Time will just add to the pile of wounds. Each time, it will open an existing wound, open a scab, and infection will add to the wound.

You must let it go. When you let your blood flow from a cut, your body will eventually scab over, heal, and then scar. You will never be the same, but you will become stronger. The strongest part of any surface is where the healing occurred. That is the same for us physically, in physical innate objects and energetically.

A baby is born as pristine as it will ever be. Life itself inflicts wounds and scars.

When you keep the poison inside of yourself, you choose the poison.

14. Silence is not golden if it requires you to hold your voice and tongue.

    Your voice is crucial to your well-being and purpose. You were born with a purpose, and voice is how you project it to the world. We have been taught disempowerment by silencing our voices.

    Do not suppress or deny your thoughts and feelings. They are the language of your soul, and your soul is here for a reason.

    Your voice matters. Your opinions matter. Your experience matters. Your desires and wants matter. Your dreams matter.

    Silence is for going inward for your own power to hear the voice of your soul. Once your soul has spoken, speak it loudly and proudly, and do not stop for anything or anyone.

15. Money can't buy happiness, but it is an external representation of your inner world.

    Money is a result.

    Money is the energy and value that you bring to the world.

    You have a special gift that the world needs and is waiting for. You were designed to live in prosperity and abundance.

    If you are lacking money, then you are not living on a solid foundation, and your world will be unstable. It is information telling you where your foundation needs support. Look at the information that it is telling you.

    If you are lacking money, then you are not aligned with yourself, your gifts, your purpose, and your place in the world. You are out of balance and it is your responsibility to get yourself back into balance and be a harmonious part of the system we all live in.

If you are living in lack of any kind, then you are disempowered and dependent. Every person is entitled to and responsible for being independent and empowered. The more money you have, the more responsibility you have to use it wisely for yourself and the world.

Like a dam, when you are greedy and hoard money, you are creating disease. Money, like oxygen, water, or blood, must continue to flow in order to be life-giving. Stagnation of the money flow cuts off the flow of life.

16. Practice makes progress not perfection.

Practice is part of the process of nature. There is a rhythm of our world, a pattern that brings us into alignment. Practice is growth, but there is no end result of perfection for us to attain.

Perfection is a concept and an ideal that varies based on each person. If you were to achieve perfection for one, it would not be acceptable to another.

The only perfection exists in alignment.

The highest vibrating frequency is alignment. Find your personal alignment and balance. Stay true to yourself. Living your life on purpose and in alignment is the reason for your being.

As I finish I need to share one last thing...

As a member of She Rises Studios (the publisher of this book) I participate in a women's networking group called Coffee Connect Create which is open to all for free on Thursdays 7am PST. Today's group talked about the challenges we faced and when we feel ready to give up, to throw in the towel and surrender. We pondered those moments when we felt overwhelmed, overextended and just depleted by the fight.

The challenge was to see how we faced that moment and became like the Phoenix and were able to RiseUP. I named my coaching business RiseUP and so this has been a theme and alignment of mine but this challenge had me face one story that I had omitted from this book.

I shared the story in the group and found support and encouragement and my vulnerability opened up others to share their own moments as well. It reminded me that we are only as alone and isolated as we choose to be because when we lead with our own vulnerability, we give others permission to be safe to follow.

I believe in universal laws and divine timing and knew that this conversation was not just random. It was my opening to be able to finish this book with this story.

I began this book with my third and final suicide attempt. In the process of telling my story I shared my first pathetic attempt as a 12 year old trying to drown myself in my own pool.

Obviously by the way I have introduced this story, it should be obvious that there was one in the middle of those attempts. Originally, I wasn't planning on sharing this story because the purpose of this book was to connect the dots of cause and effect and that traumatic experience didn't seem to fit into that objective for me at the time.

Recently, I was awoken in the middle of the night with a strong powerful message to tell this story. I will admit I felt a strong resistance.

I challenged that resistance and reviewed it with my editing team whether there was any benefit to you and my vision of this book to include it. I still wasn't fully convinced until the conversation that we had today in the group.

You have heard my story and the traumas that I have experienced with trusting women. I shared the deep losses of important people in my life and the scars it created. I shared with you the years of exhaustion, emptiness and loneliness and how it caused me to make disempowering and dysfunctional decisions, even though I am an intelligent, strong and capable woman. That is the effect of my crap.

During Covid, I became friends with a woman. Even though I was letting her into my life I wasn't letting her into my heart or my trust. I had built up walls to protect myself and that was leading to my feeling of disconnection and isolation.

I slowly began to share with her some of these stories of the abuse, of the loss, and of the tragedies of my life. We began to have fun together and slowly I was letting down my walls.

On New Year's Eve, her partner and mine had a get together to celebrate the ending of 2020. It had been a hard year for all of us. We thought this was the end of that story and we were ready to step into the newness of the next year.

I believe that Covid was a reset button for the world where we were shown the truth of ourselves, our lives and our society. The air became cleaner without a lot of air and vehicle traffic. The pace of life slowed down and we had time to breathe and think and be with ourselves. Our routines were disrupted by the social distancing. Because I believe in the power of the law of polarity I was able to see the good that came out of the devastation. Creation is born out of destruction. Chaos is the catalyst to change.

But there was also the dark side of Covid and that for a lot of us was facing those demons that had been suppressed. Or trying to continue to suppress them through over consumption of vices. Did you notice that alcohol sales were deemed a necessity? In my small community, licenses to sell alcohol brought access to our local hardware store so we didn't need to drive to the next available town.

And our group did a fine job of doing our part in the consumerism of consumption. That New Year's Eve was no exception.

The men didn't last as long as we did and so that left her and I alone. Under the influence we shared the problems that couples have, and how it was being amplified by Covid. We bonded as women and we began to feel safe around each other.

When she sat a little too close to me, I will admit that the song " I kissed a girl and I liked it" was playing in my head. I had never had a same sex encounter of any kind and in my 50's I was curious. In my mind I explored that concept and wondered what it would be like.

You know that energy can be felt by those around us, so did she pick up on my energy or did those thoughts enter my consciousness because of her thoughts, I will never know.

But when she leaned in and kissed me, I will admit I kissed her back. I felt wanted, desired and it touched on my loneliness.

For a moment.

And then the moment was done and I was back to reality. I pushed back and asked her to stop. I was in a committed relationship and I do not cheat. That was my first thought. My second thought was that my partner was asleep in the next room and that brought back memories.

My third thought was I was heterosexual and had no interest in her body parts.

I had fulfilled my curiosity. I had now kissed a girl. And yes for a moment I liked it.

But that was it for me and I clearly told her No.

I tried to pretend that it didn't happen when we met again socially but obviously it wasn't a clear no to her. She wanted to explore this further. She wanted to begin a relationship. She made additional advances on me and I had to keep saying no.

One evening, we were all together as a foursome, her partner and mine and we were enjoying an evening together outside. She left for some reason and I was tired so I excused myself and went to bed, leaving the men to enjoy further conversation and drinks. I loved seeing my partner making male friendships.

I awoke in what felt like the middle of the night by someone kissing me. I thought it was my partner who maybe found himself in the mood and was trying to wake me. I reached up and pulled him down towards me. It was in that exact split second that I realized I was not kissing my partner. I was being kissed by her. In my bed. In the privacy of my room.

Unexpected. Uninvited. Unwanted.

And every single trauma was triggered inside of me. Every moment of feeling helpless, every single date rape, every moment of betrayal by women, every moment of my voice not being heard. Everything bubbled up inside of me and I exploded.

I pushed her off and ran outside to where the men were. I was seeking support by my partner to protect me.

What he saw was a crazy, naked woman running outside. What he saw was the shame and embarrassment of me exposed in front of another man. What he felt I can only imagine but I am sure it activated and triggered every single trauma that he had suppressed in his own life.

Because instead of seeing my call for help and running to protect me, comfort me, cover me up and make me safe, he became angry, frustrated and disappointed in me.

I ran to the basement to sleep in a guest room. I felt rejected by my partner. I felt ashamed of my being seen naked in public. I felt anger at the disrespect of the woman. I felt helpless at being touched in the safety of my own home, my own room, my own bed. I felt like I would never be safe again.

When I ran to the basement, I did not run alone. I took all the pills that I had been given by the medical system and took whatever pain pills we had in the house.

I sat on the bed and spread them all out. I looked at the piles of them and a peaceful calm serenity came. It felt so right.

I took all the pills and began to write my goodbye. I remember slowly falling asleep like a puddling of fabric into the bed. I felt empty and at peace.

Then nothing.

I woke up in the emergency room of the hospital. There was a strange man sitting on a chair staring at me and saying nothing.

My partner was sitting to my right on a chair and a doctor was asking me what happened. I told him about the evening but I also downplayed everything else I was feeling and suppressing.

Did I downplay it because my partner was there? Did I downplay it because I didn't want to be a burden? Did I downplay everything and say I was good and my life was good and not share all that I was suppressing because it had become my habit, my reality and I wasn't able to face all that yet?

I don't know but my happy face mask came on. "I'm fine," I told the doctor. I have a great life. I am happy, successful and all is well in my world.

I was sent to a therapist for a few sessions. Knowing what I now know about the medical system she was doing what she thought was best but she never got me to open up. I never confided in her all that I have shared in this book.

My walls were back up and I was in full blown suppression, denial and ignore and move on mode.

The only thing that I got of value from that therapist was the knowledge that in the animal kingdom, when prey is about to be consumed by a predator they have a built in safety system that has them play dead. Their body shuts down and the predator leaves them alone. I guess in the wild, it is not safe to consume the dead so they know to go after the living for their own survival.

The therapist told me that it made sense that before I swallowed all those pills I had such a peaceful sense of calm. It felt so right and I wanted it. I wasn't angry. I wasn't desperate. I wasn't punishing anyone.

She was the first person to bring my attention to our central nervous system and how when we are overloaded and overwhelmed, our primal reflexes set in.

The reason I decided I needed to share this story is because what if that moment had been a catalyst for me to Unlearn my Crap. What if I already knew about our central nervous system and how stresses occur? What if I had done the healing work at an earlier time in my life, would

I have fought back instead of crashing when I found myself in that situation?

What if the people around me had known what I was going through? What if they knew the signs of stress and nervous breakdown, would they have intervened and got me the help I needed before I broke completely down?

What if we all knew the signs of trauma and distress? What if we all knew how our body, mind, and universal laws worked? What if personal healing was part of ongoing self care? What if we didn't feel the need to keep up appearances and not be vulnerable? What if we talked openly about our struggles and learned how to release them rather than let them build up and putrify ourselves from the inside out?

I will admit that I immediately went back into my unhealthy learned behaviour and I continued on until I broke. It would be another year or so before I lost everything and everyone, especially myself. I didn't hear the taps on the shoulder getting my attention. I didn't feel the warning signs that my body was giving me. I ignored and suppressed and avoided until I was taken completely down and out.

I know that breakdown was necessary. It was life saving for me. I had finally gotten to the place of no longer having the resources inside me to continue. I had been too strong for too long and the 2x4 of life came crashing down on me.

That breakdown saved me and my life. The clean up and healing process uncovered what was buried under all that crap. It gave me clarity. It gave me purpose.

I healed myself. I used what I had spent all my life learning to be of service to myself. I saw the connections between different modalities. Things like the universal laws that I knew about now were intimately connected to my beliefs and thoughts. I had found the connection between knowledge and integration. I had found how to use the information as tools for not just surviving but thriving.

It all just appeared before me. My brokenness allowed my intuition to be heard and accessed. I believe that our intuition is our connection to the energetic connection to the universe, to God, to source, to whatever label you want to give it. It was all just there for me, available, known and applicable.

Through this process I have learned about myself. I have learned who I am naturally. I have learned how to apply the universal laws to my everyday life and my dreams.

For the first time in my life I have discovered the feeling of personal alignment.

But that is not a constant.

Every stress, every trigger of overwhelm, every moment that I feel like I can't go on, it's too hard, I can't take another loss, another rejection, another painful step; every time I feel the "should's" of expectation that results in the feeling of inadequacy, failure, shame those thoughts of ending my life always, always reappear.

I have spent so many nights just holding on until it passes. I have had enough cognitive awareness and unlearning my crap that I know it's temporary. I know that my prefrontal cortex has been disconnected and my central nervous system has been activated.

But in those moments the call to surrender and resort to making a final decision about a temporary problem is strong.

And I have to fight for my life every single time.

I am aware that the thought has been in my mind since I was 12. I have had 3 attempts. I know that the Conditioned Responses Automatic

Programming have been established. I now need to undo and Unlearn those, every single time they come up.

Each time I get through the battle, I feel a little stronger. Each time, I feel lighter and know the process of healing has continued. I use the example of a champagne bottle. The suppressed traumas are like the pressure exerted on the champagne and even after the initial release of the bottle being opened, there remains the carbonation bubbles to be released.

Releasing our traumas and healing is like the champagne bubbles.

I am happy to say that the space between my battling those thoughts is getting wider. This past year I had to face and overcome a lot of monumental challenges. I have had to learn to let people make their own decisions even if it caused me pain. I have had to release and let go and by the words of Mel Robbins - Let Them.

I am living my boundaries and have to defend and strengthen them constantly.

I am living my values and morals and they guide my choices.

I am living aligned with who I am authentically and my choices are becoming easier to make. My choices are now either aligned or not.

I am learning to expand my choices and discern the quality of the choices that I make available to myself.

I am able to look at myself in the mirror and like what I see. That is very helpful for me as the amount of time I am now on camera with my show Unlearn the Crap & Level Up; Your Soul is Calling. I have actually learned to admire myself and like seeing myself on camera. This is BIG!

My body is still healing. I am patiently listening to it and honouring its requests. I am focused on root cause analysis and not expecting perfection or "should's".

I now give of myself freely, openly without self sacrificing. I give from a place of strength and abundance, not duty, guilt or the crap I learned.

I give to the clients I serve helping them Unlearn their Crap. I give to my family and friends. I give to my community by collaborations and mutual connections.

I now claim that I have finished my healing journey and I am aligned. I accept that alignment is a process like homeostasis and it is ongoing.

That acceptance is my freedom.

And that feeling is my wish for you.

The person I was looking for

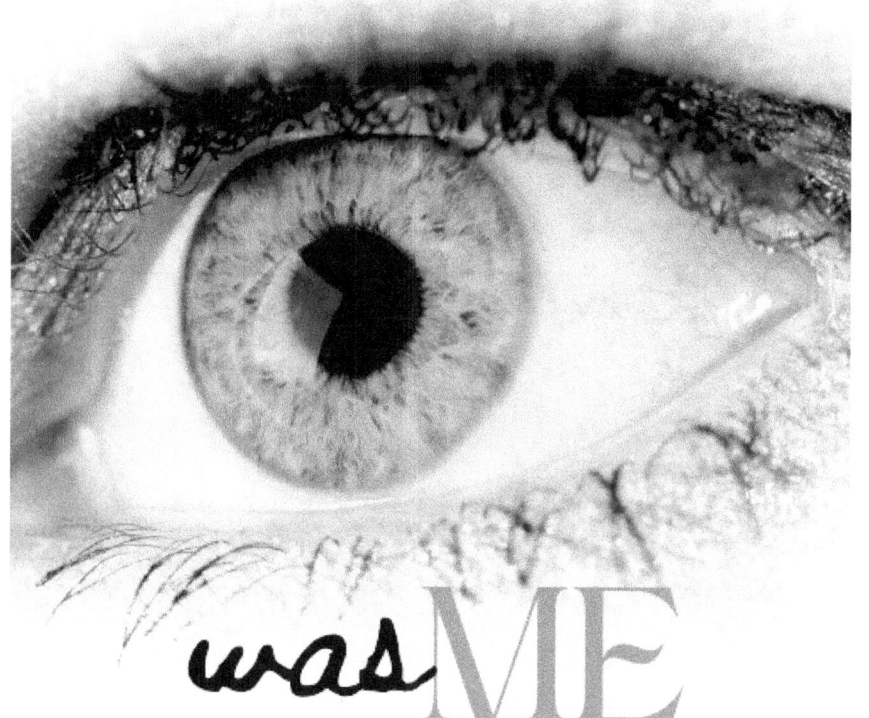

was ME

How to Work with Kathy

If you are ready to Unlearn Your Crap, I am here to help you. You do not need to go this alone. How does my process work?

I have built a process that allows you to quickly identify the crap in your way. With self awareness comes the power to choose. Healing is done with different modalities and all of them can be self administered or with a guide and mentor. My programs are designed to create immediate and lasting results. Once a trauma is released, it is gone. The healing takes the repetition of implementation to Unlearn the Crap.

I only work with clients that I am aligned with and that I know I can be of service to. I encourage you to book a call with me and let's discuss your particular situation. If I am right for you, we will find a solution that works for you.

If I am not right for you, I guarantee you that you will walk away with clarity that you can use.

Check out my website at https://kathybaldwin.me and my links at https://kathybaldwin.me/links There you will find my calendar link to book a call as well as free resources.

I encourage you to read Unlearn the Crap & Level UP Your Soul is Calling. There are the details of how to do the work involved.

I would love to have you as a subscriber to my Unlearn the Crap TV show on both FENIX TV and my YouTube Channel. This is where I have discussions with people about how to Unlearn the Crap and resources that are available for you.

I do have an Unlearn the Crap Community where we are a collection of collaborators sharing our resources and asking for what we need.

I am also a founding Managing Partner for She Wins, a division of She Rises Studios, a networking group of women entrepreneurs, business owners and professionals. My chapter is located in Canada and there are other chapters worldwide. I would love for you to join my chapter and join my online meetings, even if you can't attend the local ones (all locations are open to members) There we share resources, training, offers, networking and connection. The goal is that every woman builds a sustainable, profitable business in communities that encourage thriving.

About the Author

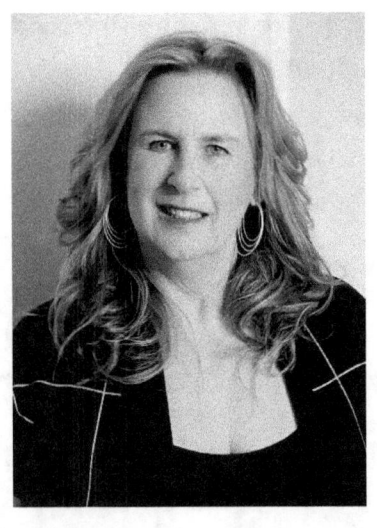

Kathy Baldwin is the author and host of Unlearn the Crap & Level UP, Your Soul is Calling, available on FENIX TV and streaming locations near you. Kathy was able to use her 40 years of experience and education in quantum physics, biology, psychology, and human behaviour to heal herself from burnout, stress, mental health, and a complete and total nervous breakdown when the medical community only offered pills and platitudes.

Her personal transformation uncovered her true authentic self and her mission and alignment. As a Life Purpose Strategist & Concierge, she implements her 4xWIN Philosophy: a Win for Her (because we all need to be first on our own list), a Win for You, a Win for our Community and most importantly a Win for the Collective Good. She is a warrior and champion for personal empowerment, believing that the power and control are moving from the minority to the majority and we have a unique purpose and mission that the world is waiting for.

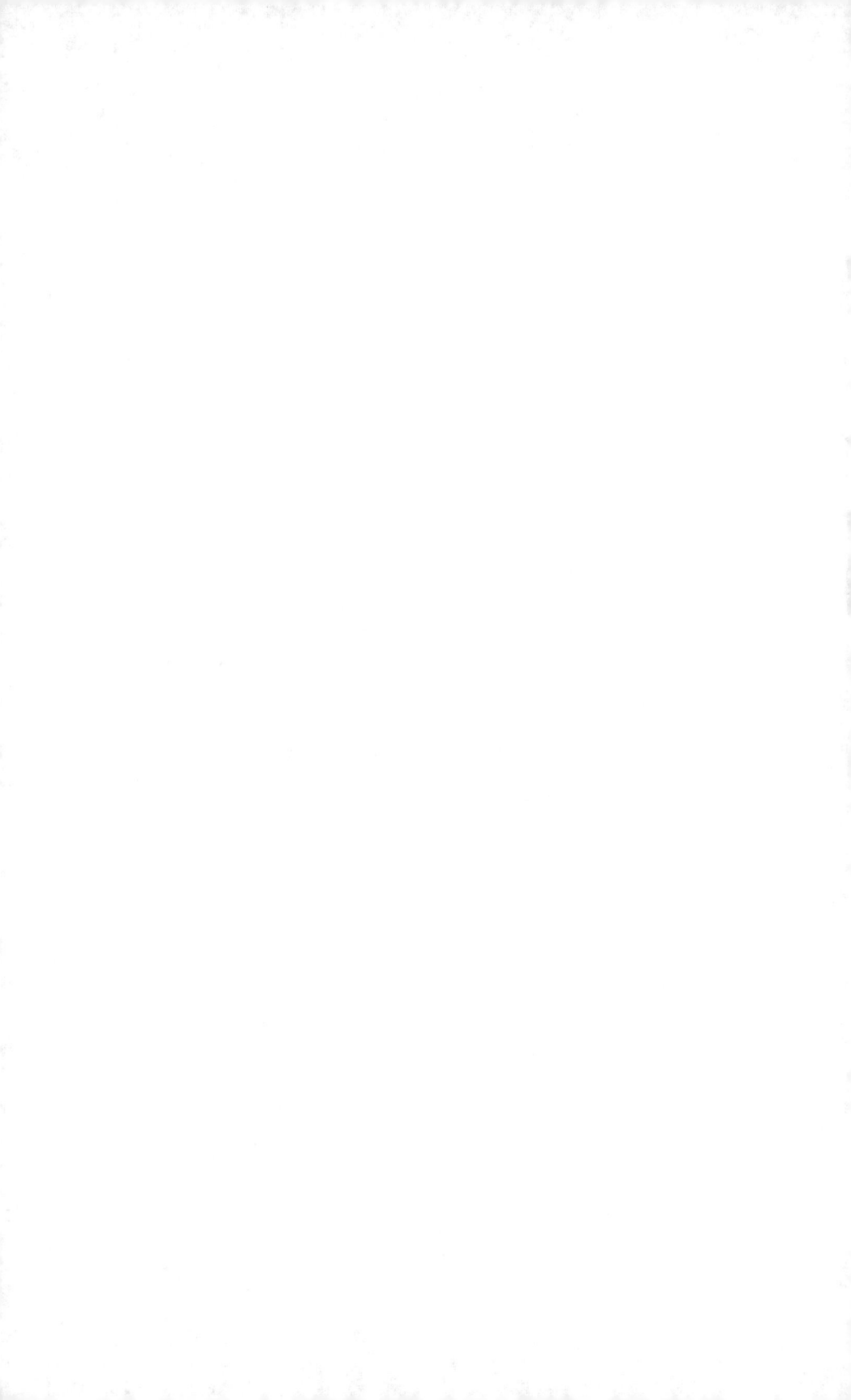

www.ingramcontent.com/pod-product-compliance
Lightning Source LLC
Chambersburg PA
CBHW071751120626
46550CB00002B/742